D0003712

Study Guide

for

The Practice of Nursing Research

Conduct, Critique, and Utilization

Fifth Edition

Study Guide

for
The Practice of Nursing Research
Conduct, Critique, and Utilization

Fifth Edition

NANCY BURNS, PhD, RN, FAAN

Jenkins Garrett Professor
Evaluation Coordinator
School of Nursing
University of Texas at Arlington
Arlington, Texas

SUSAN K. GROVE, PhD, APRN, BC, ANP, GNP

Associate Dean and Graduate Advisor
School of Nursing
University of Texas at Arlington
Arlington, Texas

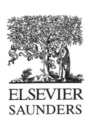

ELSEVIER
SAUNDERS

ELSEVIER
SAUNDERS

11830 Westline Industrial Drive
St. Louis, Missouri 63146

STUDY GUIDE FOR THE PRACTICE   ISBN 0-7216-0627-X
OF NURSING RESEARCH: CONDUCT,
CRITIQUE, AND UTILIZATION,
FIFTH EDITION
Copyright © 2005, 1997 by Elsevier Inc. All rights reserved.

International Standard Book Number 0-7216-0627-X

Editor: Lee Henderson
Senior Developmental Editor: Victoria Bruno
Senior Project Manager: Jeff Patterson
Cover Designer: Kathi Gosche

Printed in the United States of America

Last digit is the print number: 9 8 7 6 5 4 3 2 1

PREFACE

The amount of knowledge generated through research is rapidly escalating in the nursing field. This knowledge is critical to the promotion of quality, cost-effective, evidence-based nursing care. We recognize that learning research terminology and reading and critiquing research reports are complex and sometimes overwhelming activities. Therefore we have developed this study guide to assist you in clarifying, comprehending, analyzing, synthesizing, and applying the content presented in your textbook, *The Practice of Nursing Research: Conduct, Critique, and Utilization.*

Your study guide is organized into 29 chapters, consistent with the chapters of your textbook. Each chapter of the study guide presents you with learning exercises that require various levels of cognitive skills. These exercises are organized into the following sections: Relevant Terms, Key Ideas, Making Connections, Puzzles, Exercises in Critique, and Going Beyond. After completing the exercises for each chapter, you can review the answers in Appendix A and assess your understanding of the content. Based on your progress, you will be able to focus your study to improve your knowledge of each chapter's content. Since your learning is enhanced by exposure to a variety of visual and written experiences, we have supplemented this study guide with a CD-ROM containing bonus multiple-choice questions and an Evolve website to facilitate your comprehension of the research process.

The new **Evolve Learning Resources**, http://evolve.elsevier.com/Burns/practice, include WebLinks, an Author Index, and a Resources Appendix. The WebLinks resource provides links to related websites for each chapter. The Author Index is an alphabetical list of authors that are referenced in the textbook, and the Resources Appendix includes an extensive list of resources that can be used to enhance your learning. A list of integrative reviews of research and meta-analyses is provided to facilitate your synthesis of research knowledge on selected topics. The methodological references provide assistance in identifying and selecting methods of measurement for a study. References on theories and models from nursing and other disciplines are provided, as well as a number of references using the qualitative methodologies discussed in your text.

INTRODUCTION

This study guide was developed to accompany your textbook, *The Practice of Nursing Research: Conduct, Critique, and Utilization.* The exercises included have been designed to assist you in comprehending the content of your textbook, conducting critiques of nursing studies, using research findings to promote an evidence-based practice, and writing an initial proposal for research. It is important that you read each chapter in your text *before* completing the chapters in this study guide. First, scan the entire chapter to get an overall view of the content. Then reread the chapter with the intent of increasing your comprehension of each section. As you examine each section, pay careful attention to any terms that are defined. Underline or highlight definitions of terms in the text. If the meaning of a term is not clear to you, look up its definition in the glossary at the back of your text or in a dictionary. Highlight key ideas in each section. Examine tables and figures as they are mentioned in the text. Mark any sections that you do not fully understand. Reread these sections one sentence at a time to increase your understanding. Jot down questions to ask your instructor in class or privately.

After carefully reading a chapter in the text, use the study guide to further enhance your understanding. (Note: Each chapter in the study guide corresponds to its related chapter in your textbook.) There are six main sections to each study guide chapter: Relevant Terms, Key Ideas, Making Connections, Puzzles, Exercises in Critique, and Going Beyond.

Relevant Terms have been identified to help you become more familiar with the terms necessary to comprehend the chapter content. Knowing these terms before you attend a class lecture on the content will give you an edge in grasping the lecture ideas and doing well on course exams. In addition to completing these exercises, do not skip over terms in the chapter that are unfamiliar to you. Get in the habit of marking unfamiliar words as you read and looking up their definitions.

The **Key Ideas** section identifies information in the chapter important for you to note. The fill-in-the-blank questions will assist you in identifying important content that you might have missed in your first reading of the chapter. You may need to refer to specific sections of the text to complete some of these questions.

Making Connections between important ideas is critical to comprehending and synthesizing content. This section assists you in this process. Matching questions are frequently used for this purpose, although other strategies relevant to particular content may be used.

Puzzles, including Word Scrambles, Secret Messages, and Crossword Puzzles, are designed to help you have fun while learning. Each Word Scramble contains an important idea expressed in the chapter. The letters in each word have been rearranged. For example, "study" might be scrambled to read "tysud." Unscramble the words to decipher the message. (Hint: You may find it easier to start with the short words. Also, remember that the most commonly used letter in our language is "e.") The Secret Message puzzles are similar to the Word Scrambles, but instead of rearranging letters, you will translate each message by substituting one letter for another, thus unraveling the secret code. Finally, Crossword Puzzles have been included to help you increase your familiarity with the terms used in the chapter.

Exercises in Critique are provided to give you experience in critiquing actual studies. In some cases, brief quotes are provided with questions addressing information specific to the chapter content. Other questions will refer to Appendix B of the study guide, which includes three published studies, two quantitative and one qualitative. Critique questions related to these studies are posed in each chapter of the study guide. On completing the study guide, you can combine the critique information you have gathered to perform an overall critique of these three studies.

The **Going Beyond** section provides suggestions for further study. You might use these exercises to test your new knowledge. If the content of a particular chapter interests you, this section might direct you in learning more.

Appendix A provides the answers to the exercises in this study guide. However, we recommend that you not refer to these answers except to check your own responses to questions. You will learn more by searching for the answers on your own.

Appendix B provides reprints of the three published studies critiqued in this study guide.

Contents

CHAPTER 1

Discovering the World of Nursing Research

INTRODUCTION

Read Chapter 1 and then complete the following exercises. These exercises will assist you in learning relevant terms and understanding the framework that links nursing research with the world of nursing. The answers to these exercises are in Appendix A.

RELEVANT TERMS

Directions: Match each term below with its correct definition.

Terms

a. Abstract thinking
b. Authority
c. Concrete thinking
d. Deductive reasoning
e. Dialectic reasoning
f. Empirical world
g. Evidence-based practice

h. Inductive reasoning
i. Introspection
j. Intuition
k. Knowledge
l. Logistic reasoning
m. Nursing research

n. Operational reasoning
o. Philosophy
p. Problematic reasoning
q. Research
r. Science
s. Theory

Definitions

_____ 1. Information acquired in a variety of ways that is expected to be an accurate reflection of reality.

_____ 2. Scientific process that validates and refines existing knowledge and generates new knowledge that directly and indirectly influences nursing practice.

_____ 3. Person with expertise and power who is able to influence the opinions of others.

_____ 4. Reasoning from the specific to the general.

_____ 5. Reasoning that involves identifying a problem and the factors influencing the problem, selecting solutions to the problem, and resolving the problem.

_____ 6. Reasoning that involves the identification and discrimination among many alternatives and viewpoints and focuses on the process of debating alternatives.

_____ 7. Reasoning from the general to the specific or from a general premise to a particular situation.

_____ 8. Integrative set of defined concepts and relational statements that present a way of explaining some segment of the empirical world and can be used to describe, explain, predict, or control that segment of the world.

_____ 9. Insight or understanding of a situation or event as a whole that usually cannot be logically explained.

_____ 10. Diligent, systematic inquiry to validate and refine existing knowledge and generate new knowledge.

_____ 11. A coherent body of knowledge composed of research findings, tested theories, principles, and laws for a specific discipline.

_____ 12. Thinking oriented toward and limited by tangible things or events that are observed and experienced in reality.

_____ 13. The world experienced through our senses; the concrete portion of our existence; often called *reality*.

_____ 14. Thinking oriented toward the development of an idea without application to, or association with, a particular instance.

_____ 15. The conscientious integration of best research evidence with clinical expertise and patient values and needs in the delivery of quality, cost-effective health care.

_____ 16. The process of turning your attention inward toward your own thoughts to increase your awareness of the flow and interplay of feelings and ideas that occur.

_____ 17. Reasoning that involves examining factors that are opposites and making sense of them by merging them into a single unit or idea.

_____ 18. Reasoning that is used to break the whole into parts that can be carefully examined, as can the relationships among the parts.

_____ 19. Belief system that provides a broad, global explanation of the world.

KEY IDEAS

Directions: The knowledge generated through research is essential to provide a scientific basis for description, explanation, prediction, and control of nursing practice. Write a definition and provide an example of each of these four concepts.

1. Description:

   Example:

2. Explanation:

   Example

3. Prediction:

Example:

4. Control:

Example:

MAKING CONNECTIONS

Directions: Fill in the blanks or provide the appropriate responses.

1. List five ways of acquiring knowledge in nursing and provide an example of each.

   a.

   b.

   c.

   d.

   e.

2. Benner's (1984) book *From Novice to Expert: Excellence and Power in Clinical Practice*

   describes the importance of _____ _____ in acquiring nursing knowledge.

3. Identify Benner's five levels of experience in the development of clinical knowledge and expertise.

   a.

   b.

   c.

d.

e.

4. Nursing has _____ knowledge from other disciplines such as medicine, psychology, and sociology.

5. _____ knowledge provides a scientific basis for description, explanation, prediction, and control of nursing practice.

6. Nurses often have a "gut feeling" or "just know" when patients' conditions become very serious. This is an example of _____.

7. _____ provide knowledge based on customs and trends, such as giving a bath to hospitalized patients every morning.

8. New graduates sometimes enter internships provided by clinical agencies and are guided, supported, and educated by experienced nurses, who act as _____ to the novice nurse.

9. In the internship, new graduates are encouraged to act as _____ _____, imitating the behaviors of expert nurses.

10. Two types of logical reasoning are _____ and _____.

11. What type of reasoning do the three sentences below represent? _____

Human beings experience pain.
Babies are human beings.
Therefore babies experience pain.

12. Identify three interventions that you use frequently in your nursing practice. What is the knowledge base for each intervention?

a.

b.

c.

13. What type of knowledge is the basis for the majority of your interventions in clinical practice?

14. Identify two areas that are essential to the body of knowledge needed for nursing practice (American Nurses Association, 2003).

    a.

    b.

15. Identify two types of research that could be conducted to generate a science for nursing.

    a.

    b.

16. Identify two philosophical beliefs or values that provide a basis for the nursing profession.

17. The Seventh Report of the Joint National Committee on the Prevention, Detection, Evaluation, and Treatment of High Blood Pressure (JNC 7 Report) provides an example of a research-

    based guideline that can be used to promote _____ _____.

PUZZLES

Directions: Using the framework developed for this textbook, circle the concepts below that are directly linked to nursing research.

Philosophy

Theory

Nursing practice

Science

Abstract thought processes

Knowledge

Ways of knowing

Word Scramble

Directions: Unscramble the sentence below by rearranging the letters to form actual words. Note: You will use all the letters in every word.

Nrusgin sereahcr si rtecidly kinled ot hte rlwod fo singurn.

GOING BEYOND

Develop a framework that links research and evidence-based practice to the profession of nursing. Use the ideas and the framework presented in Chapter 1 as a basis for generating your framework. Share this framework with your instructor and classmates.

CHAPTER 2

The Evolution of Research in Nursing

INTRODUCTION

Read Chapter 2 and then complete the following exercises. These exercises will assist you in learning relevant terms and identifying the types of research conducted in nursing. The answers to these exercises are in Appendix A.

RELEVANT TERMS

Directions: Match each term below with its correct definition.

Terms

a. Correlational research
b. Critical social theory
c. Descriptive research
d. Ethnographic research
e. Experimental research
f. Grounded theory research
g. Historical research

h. Intervention research
i. Nursing process
j. Outcomes research
k. Phenomenological research
l. Philosophical inquiry
m. Problem-solving process

n. Qualitative research
o. Quantitative research
p. Quasi-experimental research
q. Research process
r. Scientific method
s. Triangulation

Definitions

_____ 1. The steps of this process include assessment, diagnosis, plan, implementation, evaluation, and modification.

_____ 2. A type of quantitative research that provides an accurate portrayal or account of characteristics of a particular individual, situation, or group; these studies are often conducted when little is known about a phenomenon.

_____ 3. Research that is considered the most objective, systematic, and controlled of the different types of quantitative research.

_____ 4. A type of qualitative research that involves describing an experience as it is lived by the person.

_____ 5. This process includes the specific steps for conducting a study.

_____ 6. Formal, objective, systematic research process to describe, test relationships, or examine cause-and-effect interactions among variables.

_____ 7. Process that involves the systematic identification of a problem, determination of goals related to the problem, identification of possible approaches to achieve those goals, implementation of selected approaches, and evaluation of goal achievement.

7

_____ 8. Procedures that scientists have used, currently use, or may use in the future to pursue knowledge.

_____ 9. A type of quantitative research that involves the systematic investigation of relationships among two or more variables.

_____ 10. Inductive research technique initially described by Glaser and Strauss that is useful in discovering what problems exist in a social scene and the processes people use to handle them, with the result being the development of a theory.

_____ 11. Systematic, subjective research methodology used to describe life experiences and give them meaning.

_____ 12. The use of multiple methods, usually quantitative and qualitative research, in the study of the same research problem.

_____ 13. A type of quantitative research that involves examining cause-and-effect relationships but has a lower level of control than experimental research.

_____ 14. Research that involves a narrative description or analysis of events that occurred in the remote or recent past.

_____ 15. A type of qualitative research that involves the use of intellectual analysis to clarify meanings, make values manifest, identify ethics, and study the nature of knowledge.

_____ 16. A type of research that was developed by the discipline of anthropology for investigating cultures through an in-depth study of the members of the culture.

_____ 17. A theory that provides the basis for research that focuses on understanding how people communicate and how they develop symbolic meanings in a society.

_____ 18. A type of research conducted to examine the end result of care or to measure the change in health status of a patient to determine if the care is cost-effective and of high quality.

_____ 19. Important new research methodology for examining the effectiveness of nursing interventions in achieving the desired outcomes in natural settings.

KEY IDEAS
Directions: Fill in the blanks or provide the appropriate responses.

1. _____ is considered the first nurse researcher.

2. *Nursing Research*, the first research journal in nursing, was first published in _____.

3. The American Nurses Association (ANA) Commission on Nursing Research established the

_____ in 1972.

4. Many national and international _____ conferences have been sponsored by Sigma Theta Tau, the international honor society for nursing since 1970.

5. The nursing research journal first published in 1978 is _____.

6. The research journal first published in 1979 is _____.

7. Identify three other research journals that were first published in 1987 or 1988.

   a.

   b.

   c.

8. _____ was the project directed by J. Horsley to promote the use of research findings in practice, the results of which were published in 1982 to 1983.

9. The *Annual Review of Nursing Research* includes:

10. The National Center for Nursing Research (NCNR) was established in _____ by the National Institutes for Health.

11. The NCNR is now called the _____.

12. The purpose of the National Institute for Nursing Research (NINR) is _____,

   _____, and _____ of information regarding basic and clinical nursing research.

13. Identify two research priorities or themes of the NINR for 2004-2005.

   a.

   b.

14. The focus during the 1980s and 1990s was the conduct of _____ research.

15. Effectiveness or outcomes research has evolved from the quality assessment and quality assurance functions that originated with the

   _____ in 1972, and more recently the peer review organizations (PROs).

16. In 1989, the _____ was established to facilitate the conduct of outcomes research.

17. For the development of an _____ practice for nursing, it is essential to conduct numerous high-quality studies.

18. In 1999, The Agency for Health Care Policy and Research (AHCPR) was reauthorized with a

    change of its name to _____.

19. Identify two future goals of the Agency for Healthcare Research and Quality (AHRQ).

    a.

    b.

20. What is the focus of *Healthy People 2010* published in 2000 by the Department of Health and Human Services?

    a.

    b.

MAKING CONNECTIONS

Directions: Match the types of processes listed below with the specific steps that follow.

Processes

a. Nursing process   b. Problem-solving process   c. Research process

Steps

_____   1. Evaluation and modification
_____   2. Knowledge of the world of nursing through clinical experience and a literature review
_____   3. Nursing diagnosis
_____   4. Methodology that includes design, sample, and methods of measurement
_____   5. Problem definition
_____   6. Assessment
_____   7. Data collection and analysis
_____   8. Outcomes and dissemination of findings

Directions: Match the following research methods with the specific types of research.

Research Methods

a. Qualitative research method
b. Quantitative research method

Research Types

_____   1.   Correlational research
_____   2.   Descriptive research
_____   3.   Ethnographic research
_____   4.   Experimental research
_____   5.   Critical social theory
_____   6.   Grounded theory research
_____   7.   Historical research
_____   8.   Phenomenological research
_____   9.   Quasi-experimental research
_____   10.   Philosophical inquiry

Directions: Match the levels of nurses' educational preparation with the research activities that each group of nurses is *primarily responsible for* according to the guidelines of the American Nurses Association (ANA).

Nurses' Educational Preparation

a. Associate degree
b. Baccalaureate degree
c. Master's degree
d. Doctoral degree (PhD or DNS)
e. Postdoctorate

Research Activities

_____   1.   Uses research findings in practice with supervision
_____   2.   Develops and coordinates funded research programs
_____   3.   Critiques studies
_____   4.   Develops nursing knowledge through research and theory development
_____   5.   Uses research findings in practice
_____   6.   Collaborates in conducting research projects
_____   7.   Conducts funded independent research projects

PUZZLES

Word Scramble

Directions: Unscramble the sentence below by rearranging the letters to form actual words. Note: You will use all the letters in every word.

Tobh tiqutaantive nad aliqutaivte sereacrh htdosem era esenstial to singnur ledkngeow. Searerch nowkdegle si deende to trconol tcosuome in urinngs actripce.

EXERCISES IN CRITIQUE

Directions: The three studies listed below are provided in Appendix B. Review the titles and abstracts of these articles. Below, match each study with the type of research conducted.

Research Types

a. Qualitative research method
b. Quantitative research method

Studies

_____ 1. Sethares & Elliott (2004)
_____ 2. Wright (2003)
_____ 3. Zalon (2004)

Directions: Review the educational, clinical, and research expertise of the authors of the three research articles in Appendix B.

1. Do Sethares and Elliott (2004) have adequate research, educational, and clinical expertise to conduct their study? Provide a rational for your response.

2. Does Wright (2003) have adequate research, educational, and clinical expertise to conduct her study? Provide a rational for your response.

3. Does Zalon (2004) have adequate research, educational, and clinical expertise to conduct her study? Provide a rational for your response.

CHAPTER 3

Introduction to Quantitative Research

INTRODUCTION

Read Chapter 3 and then complete the following exercises. These exercises will assist you in learning the steps of the quantitative research process and in identifying the different types of quantitative research (descriptive, correlational, quasi-experimental, and experimental). The answers to these exercises are in Appendix A.

RELEVANT TERMS

Directions: Match each term below with its correct definition.

Terms

a. Applied research
b. Assumptions
c. Basic research
d. Communicating research findings
e. Control
f. Data analysis
g. Data collection
h. Design
i. Framework
j. Generalization

k. Highly controlled setting
l. Interpretations of research outcomes
m. Intervention
n. Measurement
o. Methodological limitations
p. Natural setting
q. Partially controlled setting
r. Pilot study
s. Quantitative research process

t. Research problem
u. Research purpose
v. Review of literature
w. Rigor
x. Sample
y. Sampling
z. Setting
aa. Theoretical limitation
bb. Variables

Definitions

_____ 1. Formal, objective, systematic process to describe, test relationships, and examine cause-and-effect interactions among variables.

_____ 2. Location for conducting research that can be natural, partially controlled, or highly controlled by the investigator.

_____ 3. Scientific investigations conducted to generate knowledge that will directly influence clinical practice.

_____ 4. Imposition of rules by the researcher to decrease the possibility of error and increase the probability that the study's findings are an accurate reflection of reality.

_____ 5. Process of selecting a group of people, events, behaviors, or other elements that are representative of the population being studied.

_____ 6. Scientific investigations for the pursuit of "knowledge for knowledge's sake" or for the pleasure of learning.

_____ 7. A field setting that is uncontrolled by the researcher and includes real-life situations that might be examined in a study.

_____ 8. Striving for excellence in research through the use of discipline, scrupulous adherence to detail, and strict accuracy.

_____ 9. A setting for a study in which the environment is manipulated or modified in some way by the researcher.

_____ 10. Smaller version of a proposed study conducted to develop and/or refine the methodology, such as the treatment, instruments, or data collection process to be used in the larger study.

_____ 11. Artificially constructed environments that are developed for the sole purpose of conducting research.

_____ 12. The abstract, logical structure of meaning that guides the development of the study and enables the researcher to link the findings to the body of nursing knowledge.

_____ 13. The step of the research process that is generated from the problem and identifies the specific goal or aim of the study.

_____ 14. Statements that are taken for granted or are considered true, even though they have not been scientifically tested.

_____ 15. A blueprint for conducting a study that maximizes control over factors that could interfere with the study's desired outcome.

_____ 16. An area of concern in which there is a gap in the knowledge base needed for nursing practice.

_____ 17. A review and synthesis of sources (studies and theories) conducted to generate a picture of what is known and not known about a particular situation or problem of concern.

_____ 18. Terms or concepts at various levels of abstraction that are measured, manipulated, or controlled in a study.

_____ 19. A subset of a population that is selected for a particular study, the members of which are called _subjects_.

_____ 20. The process of assigning numbers to objects, events, or situations in accord with some rule.

_____ 21. Involves examining the results from data analysis, forming conclusions, exploring the significance of the findings, generalizing the findings, considering the implications for nursing practice, and suggesting further studies.

_____ 22. Involves the development and dissemination of a research report to appropriate audiences, including nurses, health professionals, health care consumers, and policy makers.

_____ 23. Limitations that restrict the abstract generalization of the findings and are reflected in the study framework.

_____ 24. Mechanism used to reduce, organize, and give meaning to data.

_____ 25. Limitations that result from weaknesses in the development of the study design, such as nonrepresentative sample, threats to design validity, single setting, limited control over the treatment, instruments with limited reliability and validity, limited control over data collection, and improper use of statistical analyses.

_____ 26. An independent variable that is manipulated to create an effect on the dependent variable.

_____ 27. The precise, systematic gathering of information relevant to the research purpose or the specific objectives, questions, or hypotheses.

_____ 28. Extending the implications of the findings from the sample that was studied to the larger population or from the situation studied to a larger situation.

KEY IDEAS

Control in Quantitative Research
Directions: Fill in the blanks in the following sentences.

1. An experimental study is conducted in a _____ _____ setting.

2. Extraneous variables need to be controlled in _____ and

   _____ research to ensure that the findings are an accurate reflection of reality.

3. _____ or _____ studies are usually uncontrolled by the researcher and conducted in natural settings.

4. _____ studies should have random selection of the sample.

5. Frequently a _____ sampling method is used in descriptive and correlational

   studies; however, a _____ sampling method might also be used.

6. A subject's home is an example of a _____ setting.

7. Laboratories or research centers are examples of _____ _____ settings.

8. Researcher control is greatest in _____ research.

9. Hospital units are _____ _____ settings that allow the researcher to control some of the extraneous variables.

10. _____ research is conducted to determine the effect of a treatment but often involves less control than experimental research.

Steps of the Research Process

Directions: Fill in the blanks or provide the appropriate responses.

1. The research process is similar to the _____ _____ and the

   _____ _____.

2. The nursing diagnosis step of the nursing process is similar to the _____ and

   _____ of the research process.

3. The plan of the nursing process is similar to the _____ of the research
   process.

4. The evaluation and modification steps of the nursing process are similar to the

   _____, _____, and

   _____ of the research process.

5. List the steps of the quantitative research process in their order of occurrence.

   Step 1:

   Step 2:

   Step 3:

   Step 4:

   Step 5:

   Step 6:

   Step 7:

   Step 8:

   Step 9:

   Step 10:

   Step 11:

   Step 12:

   Step 13:

6. What are assumptions?

7. Identify four common assumptions on which nursing studies have been based.

    a.

    b.

    c.

    d.

8. What are study limitations?

9. Identify five possible methodological limitations that you might find in published studies.

    a.

    b.

    c.

    d.

    e.

10. A small study with a limited number of subjects conducted to evaluate the effectiveness of a treatment or intervention protocol is called a _____ _____.

11. Identify five reasons for conducting a pilot study.

    a.

    b.

    c.

d.

e.

MAKING CONNECTIONS
Directions: Match the types of quantitative research listed below with the sample study titles that follow.

Research Types

a. Descriptive research
b. Correlational research
c. Quasi-experimental research
d. Experimental research

Sample Study Titles

_____ 1. Determining the Effect of a Relaxation Technique on Patients' Post-Operative Pain

_____ 2. Identifying the Incidence of HIV in Adolescents and Young Adults

_____ 3. Examining the Relationships Among Age, Gender, Knowledge of AIDS, and use of Condoms in College Students

_____ 4. Describing the Coping Strategies of Chronically Ill Men and Women

_____ 5. Determining the Effects of Position on Sacral and Heel Pressures in Hospitalized Elderly

_____ 6. Determining the Effect of Impaired Physical Mobility on Skeletal Muscle Atrophy in Laboratory Rats

_____ 7. Identifying Current Nursing Practice for Male and Female Nurses

_____ 8. Examining the Relationship Among Intensive Care Unit (ICU) Stress, Anxiety, and Recovery Rate

_____ 9. Examining the Effects of a Preadmission Self-Instruction Program on Patients' Post-operative Exercise Performance, Mood State, and Recovery Rate

_____ 10. Examining the Effects of Thermal Applications on the Abdominal Temperature of Laboratory Dogs

_____ 11. Examining the Relationships Among Hardiness, Depression, and Coping in Institutionalized Elderly

_____ 12. Determining the Incidence of Drug Abuse in Registered Nurses in Community and Hospital Settings

_____ 13. Examining the Effect of Warm and Cold Applications on the Resolution of IV Infiltrations in Hospitalized Patients

_____ 14. Determining the Stress Levels and Needs of Family Caregivers of Elderly Adults With Alzheimer's Disease

_____ 15. Examining the Effectiveness of a Breast Cancer Screening Program for Women Residing in Rural Areas

_____ 16. Identifying the Types of Care Provider (Nurse Practitioner, Physician, and Physician Assistant) Who Are Responsible for Patient Care in Primary Care Settings

_____ 17. Determining the Effectiveness of Three Wound Dressings in Patients Undergoing Heart Surgery

PUZZLES

Word Scramble

Directions: Unscramble the sentence below by rearranging the letters to form actual words. Note: You will use all the letters in every word.

Taquntiatiev sereacrh thodmes duclein cridpseitve, rrelacotiaonl, saiqu-perex-ienmtal, dna eperxmiealnt udiests.

Crossword Puzzle

Directions: Complete the crossword puzzle on the next page. Note: If the answer is more than one word, there are no blank spaces left between the words.

Across

2. Study blueprint.
4. Research method.
8. Nursing concern.
9. Null _____.
10. Type of research that seeks knowledge for knowledge's sake.
12. _____ of dependent variables in research.
14. Becker's Health Belief Model could be a study _____.
16. Location of research.
17. Strict adherence to research plan.
18. Subjects comprise this.
19. Directs a study.

Down

1. Research findings.
2. What is collected in a study?
3. Research project.
5. Known truths.
6. Study treatment is an independent _____.
7. What is reviewed prior to conducting a study?
11. Researchers _____ extraneous variables.
13. Nursing _____ to direct nursing care.
15. Practice-related studies are _____ research.

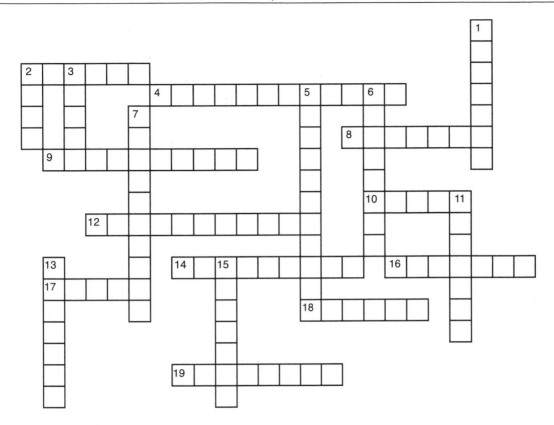

EXERCISES IN CRITIQUE

Directions: Read the research articles in Appendix B. Then identify the type of quantitative research conducted in each of the critique articles, choosing from the types of research listed below.

Research Types

a. Descriptive research
b. Correlational research
c. Quasi-experimental research
d. Experimental research
e. Qualitative research

Studies

_____   1.   Sethares & Elliott (2004)

_____   2.   Wright (2003)

_____   3.   Zalon (2004)

Directions: Now indicate whether each of the studies in Appendix B is applied or basic nursing research.

Research Types

a. Applied nursing research
b. Basic nursing research

Studies

_____   4. Sethares & Elliott (2004)
_____   5. Wright (2003)
_____   6. Zalon (2004)

GOING BEYOND

Describe two quantitative studies that you would like to conduct. Have your instructor critique the potential of conducting these studies.

1.

2.

CHAPTER 4

Introduction to Qualitative Research

INTRODUCTION

Read Chapter 4 and then complete the following exercises. These exercises will assist you in learning relevant terms and in reading and comprehending published qualitative studies. The answers for these exercises are in Appendix A.

RELEVANT TERMS

Directions: Define the following terms in your own words without looking at your text. Then check your definitions with those in the glossary of your text. Using this strategy, you can identify elements of the term that are not yet clear in your mind. Reread the relevant section of the chapter to clarify your understanding of the term.

1. Gestalt

2. Sedimented view

3. Deconstructing

4. Reconstructing

5. Ascendance to the open context

6. Embodied

7. Situated

8. Being-in-time

9. Emic approach

10. Etic approach

KEY IDEAS

Directions: Complete the following sentences.

1. Qualitative research is a way to gain insights through:

2. The reasoning process used in qualitative research involves:

3. To form new gestalts, the researcher must:

4. In qualitative research, rather than using frameworks, the study is guided by:

5. In qualitative research, rigor is associated with:

6. The purpose of phenomenological research is to:

7. Symbolic interaction theory, on which grounded theory is based, explores how:

8. According to symbolic interaction theory, reality is:

9. The word *ethnographic* means:

10. The purpose of anthropological research is:

11. The primary questions of history are:

12. Foundational inquiry studies provide analyses of:

13. In ethical inquiry, the researcher identifies:

14. According to Stevens (1989), the purpose of critical social theory is to:

MAKING CONNECTIONS

1. List three characteristics of rigor in qualitative studies.

a.

b.

c.

Directions: Match the qualitative method with the following characteristics.

Qualitative Methods

a. Phenomenological
b. Grounded theory

c. Ethnographic
d. Historical

Characteristics

_____   1.   Studies cultures
_____   2.   Studies interactions of individuals or groups
_____   3.   Studies meaning of a lived experience
_____   4.   Uses informants
_____   5.   Used to study Parse's theory
_____   6.   Studies the past
_____   7.   Gaining entry is essential
_____   8.   Uses constant comparative process
_____   9.   Develops an inventory of sources
_____   10.   Considers an experience unique to the individual

PUZZLES

Crossword Puzzle

Directions: Complete the crossword puzzle on the next page. Note: If the answer is more than one word, there are no blank spaces left between the words.

Across

1. _____ _____ mode—Strategy used to refine substantive theory
3. _____ research—A strategy of research emerging from Leininger's theory
5. Letting go of sedimented views to be open to new views
6. _____ culture—Man-made objects associated with a particular group
7. _____ research—An approach to research in which representatives from the group being studied are included in the research team
8. Theory that has its roots in the data from which it was derived
10. Striving for excellence in research
14. A branch of philosophy that deals with morality
16. Describes experiences as they are lived
18. Experiencing within a framework of time
20. _____ ethnography—Research focused on the ideas, beliefs, and knowledge that a group holds
21. _____ mode—Grounded theory research approach that provides rich detail
22. _____view—Seeing things from a specific frame of reference
23. A self within a body
24. Being shaped by your world, which constrains your ability to establish meanings

Down

2. The philosophical bases, concepts, and theories of a science
4. A way of life belonging to a designated people
9. A way of organizing data that forms new ideas
11. _____ inquiry—Uses intellectual analyses to clarify meanings, make values manifest, identify ethics, and study the nature of knowledge
12. _____ mode—Used to test the relationships of a substantive theory
13. Portrait of a people
15. _____ anthropology—Studies patterns of behavior, customs, and ways of life
17. Elements unique to each person within which that person can be understood
19. _____ mode—Identifies patterns in the life experiences of individuals

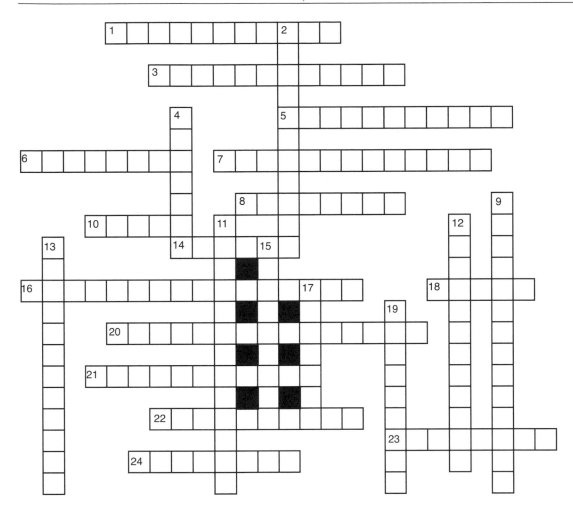

Word Scramble

Directions: Unscramble the sentence below by rearranging the letters to form actual words. Note: You will use all the letters in every word.

Cnoe oyu vaeh scadnede ot het noep txencot, ouy tancnt og kabc ot eth edai hatt het mohennopne uoy veha revsobed nac eb nese olny noe yaw.

Secret Message

Directions: Translate the secret message below by substituting one letter for another. For example, if you decide that "b" should really be "d," then "b" will be "d" every time it appears in this puzzle. Hint: Try to translate short words first to establish vowel patterns.

Gr gq apgrgayj rm slbcpqrylb rfl nfgjmqmnfw ml ufgaf lyaf osyjgryrgtc kcrfmb

gq zyqcb.

EXERCISES IN CRITIQUE

Directions: Examine the study by Wright (2003) in Appendix C and answer the following questions.

1. What is the philosophical base for Wright's study?

2. What evidence can you find that the author ascended to an open context?

3. Whose method did Wright select for her study?

4. What strategies did Wright use to achieve rigor in her study?

GOING BEYOND

Seek out a variety of published qualitative studies. Identify the philosophy on which each study is based. Does the researcher explain the philosophical base? What is the research question? How was a sample acquired? Identify the data collection and analysis strategies used. What is the outcome of the analysis process? For each study, write a paragraph summarizing information you have gathered in answering the questions above.

CHAPTER 5

Research Problem and Purpose

INTRODUCTION

Read Chapter 5 and then complete the following exercises. These exercises will assist you in critiquing problems and purposes in published studies and formulating a problem and purpose to conduct a study. The answers to these exercises are in Appendix A.

RELEVANT TERMS

Directions: Match each term below with its correct definition.

Terms

a. Approximate replication
b. Concurrent replication
c. Exact replication
d. Feasibility of study

e. Landmark study
f. Replication
g. Research problem

h. Research purpose
i. Research topic
j. Systematic replication

Definitions

_____ 1. Internal replication that involves the collection of data for the original study and its replication simultaneously to provide a check of the reliability of the original study.

_____ 2. Clear, concise statement of the specific goal or aim of the study that is generated from the problem.

_____ 3. An area of concern in which there is a gap in the knowledge base needed for nursing practice.

_____ 4. Operational replication that involves repeating the original study under similar conditions, following the original methods as closely as possible.

_____ 5. Reproducing or repeating a study to determine whether similar findings will be obtained.

_____ 6. Concept or broad problem area that provides the basis for generating numerous research problems.

_____ 7. Precise, identical duplication of the initial researcher's study to confirm the original findings.

_____ 8. Constructive replication performed under distinctly new conditions in which the researchers conducting the replication do not follow the design or methods of the original researcher; rather, the second investigative team begins with a similar problem statement but formulates new means to verify the first investigator's findings.

_____ 9. A determination made by examining the time and money commitment; the researcher's expertise; availability of subjects, facility, and equipment; cooperation of others; and the study's ethical considerations.

_____ 10. Major study generating knowledge that influences a discipline and sometimes society in general.

KEY IDEAS

Directions: Fill in the blanks or provide the appropriate responses.

1. A clearly stated research purpose includes:

   a.

   b.

   c.

2. Research problems and purposes are significant if they have the potential to generate and refine relevant knowledge that:

   a.

   b.

   c.

   d.

3. Williams' (1972) study, conducted to examine factors that contribute to skin breakdown, is

   considered a _____ study in the area of pressure ulcer prevention. Williams' study and many other studies of pressure ulcers are summarized in the document Pressure Ulcers in Adults: Prediction and Prevention, published by

   _____.

4. Studies need to be _____ to determine whether the findings are consistent from one study to another and whether they provide strong evidence for use in practice.

5. Researchers are conducting an _____ replication of a study if they are repeating the study except for using different subjects and measuring the variables with improved methods of measurement.

6. The feasibility of a research problem and purpose is determined by examining the following:

    a.

    b.

    c.

    d.

7. Three ways to determine researcher expertise is by examining the _____ prepara-

    tion, conduct of previous _____, and _____ experience in nursing
    practice.

8. Identify four sources of research problems.

    a.

    b.

    c.

    d.

9. Identify four goals of outcomes research.

    a.

    b.

    c.

    d.

10. Coping patterns, pain management, health promotion, and social support are examples of

    _____ _____ that have directed the generation of research in nursing.

11. Numerous research problems can be generated from a research topic, and a research problem

    can be used to generate numerous _____ _____.

MAKING CONNECTIONS

Directions: Match the types of research listed below with the specific purpose statements that follow.

Research Types

a. Correlational research
b. Critical social theory
c. Descriptive research
d. Ethnography

e. Experimental research
f. Grounded theory research
g. Historical research

h. Phenomenological research
i. Philosophical analysis
j. Quasi-experimental research

Purpose Statements

_____   1. To examine the evolution of the American Nurses Association's position on health care for the aged from 1935 to 1990.

_____   2. To determine how the employment, income, and coping patterns of parents changed following the birth of a low-birth-weight infant.

_____   3. To describe the lived experience of being in an intensive care unit.

_____   4. To develop a theory to describe the suffering of people with dementia of the Alzheimer type (DAT).

_____   5. To examine the relationships among spirituality, perceived social support, and income of adult children caring for their elderly parents.

_____   6. To examine the effect of a relaxation technique on perceived anxiety in working adults in high-stress jobs.

_____   7. To examine the effect of heat application on the healing rate of abdominal incisions in dogs.

_____   8. A concept analysis of caring was conducted to determine the essential elements of this significant concept in nursing.

_____   9. To examine the health practices of Hispanic women and the impact of these practices on their families.

_____   10. To determine the smoking status, alcohol dependence, and bone mineral density in postmenopausal women.

_____   11. To describe the experience of sleeplessness in depressed women.

_____   12. To determine whether social support, employment, and marital status are predictive of coping with the loss of a child.

_____   13. To examine the impact of an exercise program on muscle mass and bone mineral density in premenopausal women.

_____   14. To describe the implementation of skin care by nurses from 1850 to 1950.

EXERCISES IN CRITIQUE

Sethares and Elliot Study

Directions: Review the Sethares and Elliott (2004) research article in Appendix B and answer the following questions.

1. Identify the following parts of the problem for this study.

   a.   Significance of the problem:

   b.   Background of the problem:

   c.   Problem statement:

2. State the purpose of this study.

3. Are the problem and the purpose significant? Provide a rationale.

4. Does the purpose identify the variables, population, and setting for this study?

   a.   Identify the variables:

   b.   Identify the population:

c. Identify the setting:

5. Are the problem and purpose feasible for the researchers to study? Provide a rationale.

Wright Study

Directions: Review the Wright (2003) research article in Appendix B and answer the following questions.

1. Identify the following parts of the problem for this study.

 a. Significance of the problem:

 b. Background of the problem:

 c. Problem statement:

2. State the purpose of this study.

3. Are the problem and the purpose significant? Provide a rationale.

4. Does the purpose identify the variables, population, and setting for this study?

    a. Identify the variables:

    b. Identify the population:

    c. Identify the setting:

5. Are the problem and purpose feasible for the researchers to study? Provide a rationale.

Zalon Study

Directions: Review the Zalon (2004) research article in Appendix B and answer the following questions.

1. Identify the following parts of the problem for this study.

    a. Significance of the problem:

    b. Background of the problem:

    c. Problem statement:

2. State the purpose of this study.

3. Are the problem and the purpose significant? Provide a rationale.

4. Does the purpose identify the variables, population, and setting for this study?

   a. Identify the variables:

   b. Identify the population:

   c. Identify the setting:

5. Are the problem and purpose feasible for the researchers to study? Provide a rationale.

GOING BEYOND

1. Following the steps outlined in Figure 5-2 on p. 78 in your textbook, identify a research topic and formulate a research problem and purpose for a study of interest to you.

2. Seek feedback from your classmates and instructor in clarifying the problem and purpose you have identified.

3. Analyze whether the purpose is feasible to direct the conduct of your study by examining the time and money commitment; your expertise as a researcher; availability of subjects, facility, and equipment; cooperation of others; and the study's ethical considerations.

CHAPTER 6

Review of Relevant Literature

INTRODUCTION

Read Chapter 6 and then complete the following exercises. These exercises will assist you in reading and critiquing research reports and summarizing the findings for use in practice or for conducting research. The answers to these exercises are in Appendix A.

RELEVANT TERMS

Directions: Define the following terms in your own words without looking at your text. Then check your definitions with those in the glossary of your text. Using this strategy, you can identify elements of the term that are not yet clear in your mind. Reread the relevant section of the chapter to clarify your understanding of the term.

1. Literature review

2. Seminal study

3. Landmark study

4. Theoretical literature

5. Serials

6. Periodicals

7. Empirical literature

8. Thesis

9. Dissertation

10. Empirical knowledge

11. Primary source

12. Secondary source

13. Bibliographic database

14. Synonym

15. Complex search

KEY IDEAS

Directions: Fill in the blanks or provide the appropriate responses.

1. Provide five correct ways to complete the following statement: As a researcher, your goal is to develop a search strategy designed to:

   a.

   b.

   c.

   d.

   e.

2. List three advantages of using a library that provides access to large numbers of electronic databases.

   a.

   b.

   c.

3. Identify three elements that influence the scope of a literature review.

   a.

   b.

   c.

4. The two main types of information cited in the review of literature for research are

   _____ and _____.

5. Predominately _____ sources, not secondary sources, are used in developing a research proposal.

6. Sources for developing a literature review for a proposal can be identified through

   _____ and _____ searches.

7. Identify, in the correct order, the four steps for reviewing the literature.

   a.

   b.

   c.

   d.

8. Manual search of the literature involves examining the following:

   a.

   b.

   c.

   d.

9. What is the name of the original index for nursing literature?

10. Identify two databases commonly used by nurses to locate relevant sources.

   a.

   b.

11. The _____ is a good source of integrative
    reviews of research relevant to nursing practice.

12. Reviewing the literature requires a _____ of research sources to determine what is
    known and not known about a clinical problem.

13. What is the purpose of reference management software?

14. Identify the four common headings or content areas covered in a literature review.

    a.

    b.

    c.

    d.

15. Consider the following research problem: "Women's delay in seeking treatment for acute myocardial infarction symptoms results in higher rates of mortality and morbidity for women" (Rosenfeld, A. G. [2004]. Treatment-seeking delay among women with acute myocardial infarction. *Nursing Research*, 53[4], p. 225). What key terms would you use to direct your review of literature for this research problem?

16. Consider the following research problem: "The southern Appalachian states show a high prevalence of smoking, with associated high rates of both heart disease and cancer; yet cultural differences raise questions concerning the applicability of the most frequently used model for smoking cessation, the transtheoretical model, for smokers from this region of the county" (Macnee, C. L., & McCabe, S. [2004]. The transtheoretical model of behavior change and smokers in southern Appalachia. *Nursing Research*, 453[4], p. 243). What key terms would you use to direct your review of literature for this research problem?

17. Consider the following research problem: "Cancer-related pain often is undertreated despite the availability of effective interventions." (Vallerand, A. H., Riley-Doucet, C., Hasenau, S. M., & Templin, T. [2004]. Improving cancer pain management by homecare nurses. *Oncology Nursing Forum*, 31[4], p. 809). What key terms would you use to direct your review of literature for this research problem?

18. List three steps for limiting your search if you get too many "hits."

    a.

    b.

    c.

19. The most common sources for nursing research reports are professional journals. Identify four nursing research journals.

    a.

    b.

    c.

    d.

20. Identify three clinical journals in which research reports comprise 50% or more of the journal's content.

    a.

    b.

    c.

21. Identify the four major sections of a research report.

    a.

    b.

    c.

    d.

22. Summarizing sources to develop a literature review section for a research proposal involves

    _____, _____, _____, and _____.

23. When writing the literature review section for a research proposal, it is better to

    _____ the content of your sources than to use long direct quotes.

MAKING CONNECTIONS

Directions: Match each type of qualitative research listed below with the appropriate purpose of the literature review.

Types of Qualitative Research

a. Critical social theory
b. Ethnographic research
c. Grounded theory research

d. Historical research
e. Phenomenological research
f. Philosophical inquiry

Purpose of the Literature Review

_____ 1. Compare and combine findings from the study with the literature to determine current knowledge of a phenomenon.

_____ 2. Review literature to develop study questions; the literature is a source of data in the study.

_____ 3. Review literature to raise philosophical questions and seek answers in analyzing a variety of sources.

_____ 4. Compare and combine study findings with existing literature to determine current knowledge of a social situation.

_____ 5. Review the literature to provide a background for conducting the study, as in quantitative research.

_____ 6. Use the literature to explain, support, and extend the theory generated in the study.

Directions: Theoretical and empirical literature are included in the literature review of a published study. Consider the sources listed below; then place a "T" next to the theoretical sources and an "E" next to those sources that are empirical.

Theoretical and Empirical Literature

_____ 1. Lazarus and Folkman's *Theory of Coping*

_____ 2. Abstracts from a research conference

_____ 3. Theses

_____ 4. Watson's *Philosophy of Human Caring*

_____ 5. Orem, D. E. (1991). *Nursing: Concepts of practice* (4th ed.). St. Louis: Mosby.

_____ 6. Giuffre, M., Heidenreich, T., and Pruitt, L. (1994). Rewarming cardiac surgery patients: Radiant heat versus forced warm air. *Nursing Research*, *43*(3), 174-178.

_____ 7. Treloar, D. M. (1994). The effect of nonnutritive sucking on oxygenation in healthy, crying full-term infants. *Applied Nursing Research*, *7*(2), 52-58.

_____ 8. Dissertations

_____ 9. von Bertalanffy, L. (1968). *General systems theory*. New York: Braziller.

_____   10.   Lewin's Change Theory

_____   11.   Koniak-Griffin, D. (1994). Aerobic exercise, psychological well-being, and physical discomforts during adolescent pregnancy. *Research in Nursing Health*, *17*(4), 253-263.

Directions: A literature review includes mainly primary sources rather than secondary ones. Label the sources listed below with a "P" if they are primary or an "S" if they are secondary.

Primary and Secondary Sources

_____   1.   Integrated review of research

_____   2.   Dissertations

_____   3.   Theses

_____   4.   Textbooks

_____   5.   Summary of theoretical and empirical sources

_____   6.   Study published in *Applied Nursing Research*

Exercises in Critique

Directions: Review the three articles in Appendix B; then answer the following questions.

1. In the nursing field, the most common way to cite a reference is by using the format of the American Psychological Association (APA). Knowing the different parts of a reference citation will assist you in locating and recording sources for a formal paper. The following source is presented in APA format:

Sethares, K. A., & Elliott, K. (2004). The effect of a tailored message intervention on heart failure readmission rates, quality of life, and benefit and barrier beliefs in persons with heart failure. *Heart & Lung*, *33*(4), 249-260.

a.   What is *Heart & Lung* in this reference?

b.   What is "2004" in this reference?

c.   What is "33" in this reference?

d.   What is "249-260" in this reference?

   e. What is "(4)" in this reference?

   f. Who are the authors of this article?

2. Write a proper reference citation for the Zalon (2004) article using APA format.

3. Carefully review the three reference citations listed below. Are they complete? If not, indicate what is missing.

   a. Wright, V. L. (1994). *Archives of Psychiatric Nursing*, *17*(4).

   b. McNee, C. L., & McCabe, S. (2004). The transtheoretical model of behavior change and smokers in southern Appalachia. *Nursing Research*, (4).

   c. Rosenfeld, A. G. Treatment-seeking delay among women with acute myocardial infarction: Decision trajectories and their predictors. *Nursing Research*, 225-236.

4. What are the titles of the literature review sections of the three articles in Appendix B?

   a. Sethares and Elliott (2004):

   b. Wright (2004):

   c. Zalon (2004):

5. Are relevant studies identified and described in Zalon's (2004) study? Give examples of two studies that are cited in the study's literature review.

6. Are relevant theories identified and described in the Sethares and Elliott (2004) study? Identify a theoretical source that is cited in the study's literature review.

7. In Zalon's (2004) references, is the source by Rubin and Hotopf (2002) a primary or secondary source?

8. Are the references in Zalon's (2004) study current? Provide a rationale.

9. Does the literature review in the Sethares and Elliott (2004) study present the current knowledge base for the research problem? Provide a rationale.

10. Are relevant studies identified and described in the Sethares and Elliott (2004) study? Give examples of two studies that are cited in the literature review of the article.

11. Are relevant theories identified and described in the Zalon (2004) study? Identify one theoretical source that is cited in the study's literature review.

12. a.   In the Zalon (2004) study, is the source by Barsevick, Pasacreta, and Orsi (1995) a primary or secondary source?

   b.   Is the source by Devine et al (1999) a primary or secondary source?

13. Are the references in the Sethares and Elliott (2004) study current? Provide a rationale.

14. Does the literature review of Zalon's (2004) study provide the current knowledge base of the problem examined in this study? Provide a rationale.

15. Are relevant studies identified and described in the Wright (2003) study? Give examples of two studies that are cited in the study's literature review.

16. Are relevant theories identified and described in the Wright (2003) study? Identify two theoretical sources that are cited in the study's literature review.

17. a.   In Wright's (2003) study, is the source by Davis (1997) a primary or secondary source?

    b.   Is the source by Brisbane and Womble (1985) a primary or secondary source?

18. Are the references in Wright's (2003) study current? Provide a rationale.

19. Does the literature review in Wright's (2003) study provide a current knowledge base for the research problem examined in the study?

GOING BEYOND

1. Identify a problem in clinical practice and conduct a summary of the research literature on this topic.

2. Search the literature for relevant research sources for the problem you identified above. Has an integrative review been done on this topic? Review the list of integrated reviews of nursing research and meta-analyses provided in Appendix C of this study guide.

3. Locate relevant studies in your university library.

4. Read each study and identify the steps of the research process.

5. Outline key information from each study, including the study purpose, framework, sample size, design, results, and findings.

6. Critique the quality of each study.

7. Write a description of each research report and critique the quality of the report.

8. Write a summary paragraph that indicates what is known and not known about your clinical problem.

9. Ask your instructor to evaluate your review of the research literature.

CHAPTER 7

Frameworks

INTRODUCTION

Read Chapter 7 and then complete the following exercises. These exercises will assist you in learning relevant terms and identifying and critiquing frameworks in published studies. The answers to these exercises are in Appendix A.

RELEVANT TERMS

Directions: Define the following terms in your own words without looking at your text. Then check your definitions with those in the glossary in your text. Using this strategy, you can identify elements of the term that are not yet clear in your mind. Reread the relevant section of the chapter to clarify your understanding of the term.

1. Abstract

2. Asymmetrical relationship

3. Concept

4. Concept analysis

5. Concept derivation

6. Concept synthesis

7. Conceptual definition

8. Concrete

9. Conceptual map

10. Conceptual model

11. Conceptual definition

12. Concurrent

13. Contingent relationship

14. Construct

15. Curvilinear relationship

16. Denotative definition

17. Deterministic relationship

18. Direction of a relationship

19. Effect size

20. Existence statement

21. Framework

22. General proposition

23. Hierarchical statement

24. Hypotheses

25. Intervening variable

26. Linear relationship

27. Mediating variable

28. Necessary relationship

29. Negative relationship

30. Positive relationship

31. Probability statement

32. Relational statement

33. Research tradition

34. Proposition

35. Scientific theory

36. Sequential

37. Specific proposition

38. Strength of a relationship

39. Substantive theory

40. Substitutable relationship

41. Substruction

42. Sufficient relationship

43. Symmetrical relationship

44. Tendency statement

45. Tentative theory

46. Theory

47. Theoretical substruction

48. Variable

KEY IDEAS
Directions: Fill in the blanks or complete the following sentences.

1. We use theories to:

2. Testing a theory involves:

3. _____ _____ are not generally considered testable.

4. Research is based on _____.

5. The strength of a relationship is sometimes described with the term _____

   _____.

6. Research findings are interpreted in terms of the _____.

7. In a framework, all _____ should be defined.

8. Concepts in conceptual models are referred to as _____.

9. A _____ is more specific than a concept and is defined so that it is measurable.

10. The _____ of a theory are tested through research.

11. Statements at the lowest level of abstraction are referred to as _____.

12. The purpose of a conceptual map is to:

13. A conceptual map includes:

14. An organized program of research designed to build a body of knowledge related to a particular

    conceptual model is referred to as a _____ _____.

Making Connections

Directions: Match each term below with its definition.

Terms

a. Theory
b. Concept
c. Conceptual model

d. Variable
e. Statement
f. Conceptual map

g. Framework
h. Construct
i. Hypothesis

Definitions

_____   1. Broadly explains phenomena of interest
_____   2. The basic element of a theory
_____   3. Expresses a claim important to a theory
_____   4. Graphically shows interrelations among concepts
_____   5. Integrated set of defined concepts and statements
_____   6. Statement expressed at low level of abstraction
_____   7. Provides general meanings of terms
_____   8. Defines a term so that it is measurable
_____   9. Presents portions of a theory to be tested in a study

PUZZLES

Word Scramble
Directions: Unscramble the sentence below by rearranging the letters to form actual words. Note: You will use all the letters in every word.

Amyn tusidse rea duirqere ot diavelat lal fo eht tesnamtets ni a yrehto.

Secret Message
Directions: Translate the secret message below by substituting one letter for another. For example, if you decide that "i" should really be "g," then "i" will be "g" every time it appears in this puzzle. Hint: Try to translate short words first to establish vowel patterns.

Aqw pggf vq fgvgtokpg nkpmu coqpi vjg eqpegrvwcn fghkpkvkqpu, vjg

xctkcdngu kp vjg uvwfa, cpf vjg tgncvgf ogcuwtgogpv ogvjqfu.

Crossword Puzzle
Directions: Complete the crossword puzzle on the next page. Note: If the answer is more than one word, there are no blank spaces left between the words.

Across

1. Not considered testable through research.
4. Framework with ideas not fully developed.
6. Portion of a theory to be tested in a study.
7. Specific statement expressed at lowest level of abstraction.
11. Focus of Orem's Model.
12. Expression of an idea apart from any specific instance.
13. Term in which numerical values vary from one instance to another.
14. An organized program of research designed to build a body of knowledge related to a particular conceptual model.

Down

1. Ideas concerned with realities or actual instances.
2. Process of determining the truth of a relational statement.
3. Developed to explain which concepts contribute to or partially cause an outcome.
5. Used to describe, explain, predict, and/or control a phenomenon.
8. Statement found in theories.
9. Clarifies the type of relationship that exists between or among concepts.
10. Focus of Roy's Model.

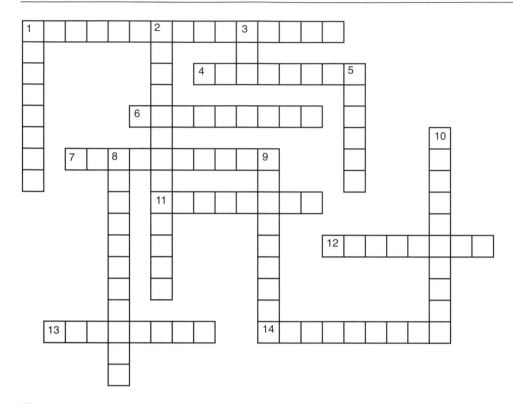

EXERCISES IN CRITIQUE

Directions: Examine the framework of Zalon's (2004) study provided in Appendix B.

1. List the concepts in the study.

2. State the definition of each concept as defined by the author(s). Are the definitions clear and adequate? If not, identify the inadequacies.

3. List the variables used in the study.

4. Identify the concept(s) with which each study variable is associated.

5. Describe the method used to measure each variable.

6. Complete the following table by listing each concept, the related variable(s), and the measurement method(s).

Concept	Variable(s)	Measurement Method(s)

7. Compare the measurement method for each variable with its associated concept and conceptual definition. Is each measurement method consistent with its associated concept and conceptual definition? If not, what are the inconsistencies?

8. List the statements expressed within the Zalon (2004) study. Then underline the concepts included in each statement. Are all of the study concepts included within each statement? Provide a map of each statement.

9. State the propositions being tested in the study and the related hypotheses or research questions.

10. Are the statements tested by the study design? How?

11. Is the framework expressed as a conceptual map? Are all of the concepts in the study included in the map? Are all of the statements you identified included in the map? If there is no map, develop one and draw it here.

12. Does the author provide statements for each linkage between concepts shown on the map? Does the author provide references from the literature to support the linkages? If so, list the references for each linkage.

13. Develop a short summary paragraph describing the strengths and weaknesses of the framework of the Zalon (2004) study.

Going Beyond

Critique the framework of the Sethares and Elliott (2004) study in Appendix B using questions 1 through 13 of the Exercises in Critique section above. Ask your instructor to review your critique.

CHAPTER 8

Objectives, Questions, and Hypotheses

INTRODUCTION

Read Chapter 8 and then complete the following exercises. These exercises will assist you in critiquing objectives, questions, hypotheses, and variables in published studies. The content will also help you in developing research objectives, questions, or hypotheses for a study and in conceptually and operationally defining the variables to be studied. The answers to these exercises are in Appendix A.

RELEVANT TERMS

Directions: Match each term below with its correct definition.

General Concepts

a. Hypothesis
b. Research objective
c. Research question
d. Variables

Definitions

_____ 1. Clear, concise, declarative statements that are expressed in the present tense and are used to direct the conduct of a study.

_____ 2. Concepts at various levels of abstraction that are measured, manipulated, or controlled in a study.

_____ 3. A formal statement of the expected relationship(s) between two or more variables in a specified population.

_____ 4. Concise interrogative statement developed to direct a study; focuses on description of variables, examination of relationships among variables, and determination of differences between two or more groups.

Directions: Match each type of hypothesis below with its correct definition.

Types of Hypotheses

a. Associative hypothesis
b. Causal hypothesis
c. Complex hypothesis
d. Directional hypothesis

e. Nondirectional hypothesis
f. Null hypothesis
g. Research hypothesis
h. Simple hypothesis

Definitions

_____ 1. Hypothesis stating the relationship (associative or causal) between two variables.

_____ 2. Alternative hypothesis to the null hypothesis, which states that a relationship exists between two or more variables.

_____ 3. Hypothesis stating that a relationship between two variables where one variable (independent variable) is thought to cause or determine the presence of the other variable (dependent variable).

_____ 4. Hypothesis stating that a relationship exists but does not predict its exact nature.

_____ 5. Hypothesis predicting the relationships (associative or causal) among three or more variables.

_____ 6. Hypothesis stating a relationship in which variables or concepts that occur or exist together in the real world are identified; when one variable changes, the other variable changes.

_____ 7. Hypothesis stating the specific nature of the interaction or relationship between two or more variables.

_____ 8. Hypothesis stating that no relationship exists between the variables being studied.

Directions: The following terms are related to variables. Match each term with its correct definition.

Types of Variables

a. Conceptual definition
b. Demographic variable
c. Dependent variable

d. Extraneous variable
e. Independent variable
f. Operational definition

Definitions

_____ 1. Definition that provides a variable or concept with a connotative (abstract, comprehensive, theoretical) meaning.

_____ 2. Variable that exists in all studies and can affect the measurement of study variables and the relationships among these variables.

_____   3. Definition that describes how variables or concepts will be measured or manipulated in a study.

_____   4. Response, behavior, or outcome that is predicted or explained in research; changes in this variable are presumed to be caused by the independent variable.

_____   5. Treatment or experimental activity that is manipulated or varied by the researcher to create an effect on the dependent variable.

_____   6. Characteristics or attributes of subjects that are collected to describe the sample.

KEY IDEAS

Directions: Fill in the blanks or provide the appropriate responses.

1. The research problem and purpose provide a basis for the formulation of specific

   _____, _____, or _____ to direct the conduct of a study.

2. Causal relationships identify a cause-and-effect interaction between two or more variables,

   which are referred to as _____ and _____ variables.

3. Terms such as _less_, _more_, _increase_, and _decrease_ indicate the _____ of relationships in hypotheses.

4. H_0 is the symbol used to represent a _____ _____.

5. A testable hypothesis is one that:

6. Other terms that are used for the independent variable include:

7. Other terms that are used for the dependent variable include:

8. Qualitative studies sometimes involve the investigation of _____ instead of variables.

9. Variables that are not recognized until the study is in process or are recognized before the study

   is initiated but cannot be controlled are referred to as _____ variables.

10. _____ variables are a type of extraneous variable that make up the setting where the study is conducted.

11. The demographic variables, such as subjects' age, gender, and ethnic background, are analyzed

to provide a picture of the sample, or the _____ _____.

MAKING CONNECTIONS

Directions: Listed below are types of hypotheses. Following that list are ten specific sample hypotheses. Identify each specific hypothesis by indicating which terms apply to it. Hint: Four terms are needed to identify each hypothesis. The correct answer for hypothesis 1 is provided as an example.

Types of Hypotheses

a. Associative
b. Causal
c. Complex
d. Direction

e. Nondirectional
f. Null
g. Research
h. Simple

Sample Hypotheses

b, c, d, g 1. Relaxation therapy is more effective than standard care in decreasing pain perception and use of pain medications in adults with chronic arthritic pain.

_____ 2. Age, family support, and health status are related to the self-care abilities of nursing home residents.

_____ 3. Heparinized saline is no more effective than normal saline in maintaining the patency and comfort of a heparin lock.

_____ 4. Poor health status is related to decreasing self-care abilities in institutionalized elderly adults.

_____ 5. Low-back massage is more effective in decreasing perception of low-back pain than no massage in patients with chronic low-back pain.

_____ 6. Healthy adults involved in a diet and exercise program have lower low-density lipoprotein (LDL), higher high-density lipoprotein (HDL), and lower cardiovascular risk levels than adults not involved in the program.

_____ 7. Time on the operating table, diastolic blood pressure, age, and preoperative albumin levels are related to development of pressure ulcers in hospitalized elderly adults.

_____ 8. There are no differences in complications or incidence of phlebitis in heparin locks changed every 72 hours and those locks left in place up to 168 hours.

_____ 9. Nurses' perceived work stress, internal locus of control, and social support are related to their psychological symptoms.

_____ 10. Cancer patients with chronic pain who listen to music with positive suggestion of pain reduction have less pain than those who do not listen to music.

11. Rewrite hypothesis 2 above as a directional hypothesis.

12. Rewrite hypothesis 5 above as a null hypothesis.

Directions: Match the types of variables below with the sample variables that follow.

Types of Variables

a. Demographic variable   b. Dependent variable   c. Independent variable

Sample Variables

_____   1.   Age
_____   2.   Perception of pain
_____   3.   Exercise program
_____   4.   Gender
_____   5.   Length of hospital stay
_____   6.   Incidence of phlebitis
_____   7.   Relaxation therapy
_____   8.   Low-back massage
_____   9.   Educational level
_____   10. Postoperative pain
_____   11. Ethnic background
_____   12. Marital status

EXERCISES IN CRITIQUE: OBJECTIVES, QUESTIONS, OR HYPOTHESES AND STUDY VARIABLES

Sethares and Elliott Study
Directions: Review the Sethares and Elliott (2004) research article in Appendix B and answer the following questions.

1. Are objectives, questions, or hypotheses stated in the study? Identify them.

2. Are objectives, questions, and hypotheses appropriate and clearly stated? Provide a rationale.

3. List the variables in this article and identify the type of each variable (independent, dependent, or research).

4. Identify the conceptual and operational definitions for the independent variable: tailored message for patients with HF.

5. Identify the demographic variables in this study.

Wright Study

Directions: Review the Wright (2003) research article in Appendix B and answer the following questions.

1. Are objectives, questions or hypotheses stated in the study? Identify them.

2. Are objectives, questions or hypotheses appropriate and clearly stated? Provide a rationale.

3. List the variables in this article and identify the type of each variable (independent variable, dependent variable, or research variable or concept).

4. Identify the conceptual and operational definitions for the research concept: lived experience of spirituality of recovery from substance abuse.

5. Identify the demographic variables in this study.

Zalon Study

Directions: Read the Zalon (2004) research article in Appendix B and answer the following questions.

1. Are objectives, questions or hypotheses stated in the study? Identify them.

2. Are objectives, questions or hypotheses appropriate and clearly stated? Provide a rationale.

3. List the variables in this article and identify the type of each variable (independent, dependent, or research).

4. Identify the conceptual and operational definitions for the dependent variable: depression.

5. Identify the demographic variables in this study.

GOING BEYOND

1. Develop specific objectives, questions, or hypotheses to direct a proposed study.

2. Link the objectives, questions, or hypotheses developed to the study purpose and framework.

3. Identify the variables to be studied and develop conceptual and operational definitions for each variable.

CHAPTER 9

Ethics in Research

INTRODUCTION

Read Chapter 9 and then complete the following exercises. These exercises will assist you in understanding the ethical aspects of studies. The answers for these exercises are in Appendix A.

RELEVANT TERMS

Directions: Match each term below with its correct definition.

Terms

a. Anonymity
b. Benefit-risk ratio
c. Breach of confidentiality
d. Complete institutional review
e. Confidentiality
f. Covert data collection
g. Declaration of Helsinki
h. Deception
i. Department of Health and Human Services Protection of Human Subjects Regulations

j. Ethical principles
k. Exempt from institutional review
l. Expedited institutional review
m. Food and Drug Administration Protection of Human Subjects Regulations
n. Health Insurance Portability and Accountability Act (HIPAA)
o. Human rights

p. Informed consent
q. Institutional review
r. Nontherapeutic research
s. Nuremberg Code
t. Privacy
u. Right to fair treatment
v. Right to protection from discomfort and harm
w. Right to self-determination
x. Scientific misconduct
y. Therapeutic research
z. Voluntary consent

Definitions

_____ 1. Claims and demands that have been justified in the eyes of an individual or by the consensus of a group of individuals and are protected in research.

_____ 2. Condition in which a subject's identity cannot be linked, even by the researcher, with his or her individual responses.

_____ 3. Agreement by a prospective subject to voluntarily participate in a study after he or she has assimilated essential information about the study.

_____ 4. Research conducted to generate knowledge for a discipline; the results might benefit future patients but will probably not benefit the research subjects.

_____ 5. Occurs when subjects are unaware that research data are being collected because the investigator does not inform or misinforms them about the study.

_____ 6. Process of examining studies for ethical concerns by a committee of peers.

_____ 7. Ethical document that was adopted in 1964 and revised in 1975 by the World Medical Assembly to differentiate therapeutic research from nontherapeutic research.

_____ 8. Studies that have no apparent risks for the research subjects require this type of institutional review.

_____ 9. Ratio considered by researchers and reviewers of research as they weigh potential benefits and risks in a study to promote the conduct of ethical research.

_____ 10. Principles of respect for persons, beneficence, and justice, which are relevant to the conduct of research.

_____ 11. Management of private data in research in such a way that subjects' identities are not linked with their responses.

_____ 12. Ethical code of conduct developed in 1949 that contains rules to guide the investigators in conducting research ethically.

_____ 13. Freedom of an individual to determine the time, extent, and general circumstances under which private information will be shared with or withheld from others.

_____ 14. This human right is based on the ethical principle of respect for persons, which states that humans are capable of controlling their own destinies.

_____ 15. Occurs when the subject is actually misinformed about a study for the purposes of the research; the classic example is the Milgram (1963) study.

_____ 16. Occurs when a researcher, by accident or direct action, allows an unauthorized person to gain access to raw data of a study.

_____ 17. A human right, based on the principle of justice, that states the selection of subjects and their treatment during the course of a study should be fair.

_____ 18. A human right, based on the principle of beneficence, that states subjects should be protected from physical, emotional, social, and economic discomfort and harm.

_____ 19. This means that the prospective subject has decided to take part in a study of his or her own volition without coercion or any undue influence.

_____ 20. Research that provides a patient with an opportunity to receive an experimental treatment that may have beneficial results.

_____ 21. The governmental act that established the category of protective health information, which allows covered entities, such as health plans, health care clearinghouses, and health care providers, to transmit health information to others in only certain situations.

_____ 22. Studies that have some risks, viewed as minimal, require this type of institutional review.

_____ 23. Involves such practices as fabrication, falsification, or forging of data; dishonest manipulation of the study design or methods; and plagiarism.

_____ 24. Government regulations developed to protect the rights and welfare of human subjects involved in research conducted or supported by the U.S. Department of Health and Human Services.

_____ 25. Studies that have greater than minimal risks must receive this type of review.

_____   26.   Government regulations developed to protect the rights, safety, and welfare of subjects involved in clinical investigations regulated by the Food and Drug Administration (FDA).

KEY IDEAS

Directions: Fill in the blanks or provide the appropriate responses.

1. List the three ethical principles that are relevant to the conduct of research involving human subjects.

   a.

   b.

   c.

2. List three examples of legally or mentally incompetent subjects.

   a.

   b.

   c.

3. Children 7 years of age and older are relatively _____ (*competent* or *incompetent*) to give permission to be part of a study.

4. All children must be given the opportunity to _____ to participation in research.

5. Levine (1986) identified two approaches that families, guardians, researchers, or Institutional Review Boards (IRBs) may use when making decisions on behalf of legally and mentally incompetent individuals, such as those with senile dementia of the Alzheimer type (SDAT): (1) best interest standard and (2) substituted judgment standard. Describe what these approaches involve.

   a.   Best interest standard

   b.   Substituted judgment standard

6. Maintaining confidentiality is more difficult in _____ (*quantitative* or *qualitative*) research.

7. Identify the elements of informed consent.

    a.

    b.

    c.

    d.

8. Identify five types of information that must be included on the consent form.

    a.

    b.

    c.

    d.

    e.

9. _____ consent means that the prospective subject with hypertension has decided, based on his or her own volition without coercion or any undue influence, to take part in a study focused on the management of hypertension.

10. In hospitals, before a study is conducted, it must be reviewed by a committee of peers, called

    an _____ _____ _____.

11. Identify mechanisms by which consent may be documented.

    a.

    b.

    c.

12. Fabrication of data in a study is an example of _____ _____.

13. The Office of Research Integrity (ORI) is responsible for:

14. Identify four issues that are relevant in addressing the problem of scientific misconduct.

   a.

   b.

   c.

   d.

15. The three levels of institutional review of research are:

   a.

   b.

   c.

16. Identify two important questions that need to be addressed related to the use of animals in research.

   a.

   b.

17. Over 700 institutions conducting health-related research with animals have sought accreditation

   by the _____ to ensure the humane treatment of animals in research.

18. How do you assess the benefit-risk ratio of a published study?

19. You are using school-age children in your study to implement a treatment to promoted improved weight management. What type of consent must be obtained and from whom to conduct this study?

20. Social security numbers are an example of _____ _____ _____ under HIPAA.

MAKING CONNECTIONS

Directions: Match the levels of discomfort or harm listed below with the examples that follow.

Levels of Discomfort or Harm

a. No anticipated effects
b. Temporary discomfort
c. Unusual levels of temporary discomfort

d. Risk of permanent damage
e. Certainty of permanent damage

Examples

_____ 1. Collecting an additional blood sugar sample from a diabetic patient.

_____ 2. Reviewing patient records for medical diagnoses, complications, and length of hospital stay.

_____ 3. Confining a patient to bed for 10 days to determine the impact on muscle strength, joint mobility, and bone density.

_____ 4. Collecting data on a person's child abuse and drug use behavior.

_____ 5. Data collected during the Nazi medical experiments.

_____ 6. Involving sedentary females over 45 years of age in an exercise program with progressive increases in the strenuousness of the exercises.

_____ 7. Completing an anonymous survey on satisfaction with a health care agency's services.

_____ 8. Examining the effect of new drugs that may have some very serious side effects.

_____ 9. The conduct of the Tuskegee syphilis study and the continuation of the study for several years after the treatment for syphilis was identified.

_____ 10. Studying the emotional impact of experiencing a rape.

Directions: Match the unethical studies listed below with the correct descriptions.

Unethical Studies

a. Jewish chronic disease hospital study
b. Nazi medical experiments

c. Tuskegee syphilis study
d. Willowbrook study

Descriptions

_____ 1. Subjects were exposed to freezing temperatures, high altitudes, poisons, untested drugs, and experimental operations.

_____ 2. Study was conducted to determine the natural course of syphilis in the adult black male.

_____ 3. Subjects were deliberately infected with the hepatitis virus.

_____ 4. Subjects were frequently killed or sustained permanent physical, mental, or social damage during these studies.

_____ 5. Subjects did not receive penicillin even after it was identified as an effective treatment for their disease.

_____ 6. The purpose of this study was to determine the patients' rejection responses to live cancer cells.

_____ 7. The subjects in this study were institutionalized mentally retarded children.

_____ 8. These experiments resulted in the development of the Nuremberg Code.

_____ 9. The subjects were injected with live cancer cells without their knowledge.

_____ 10. This study continued until 1972, when an account of the study appeared in the Washington Star and public outrage demanded the study be stopped.

PUZZLES

Crossword Puzzle

Directions: Complete the crossword puzzle below. Note: If the answer is more than one word, there are no blank spaces left between the words.

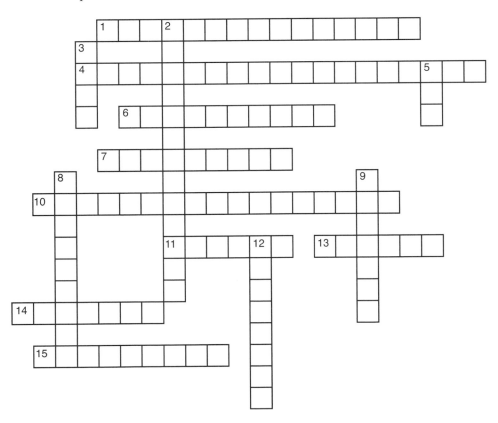

Across

1. Keeping data private.
4. Agency evaluation of a study to protect potential subjects.
6. Subjects who can legally choose whether or not to participate in a study are _____.
7. Code developed after World War II.
10. Controlling your own fate.
11. Focuses on human rights of research.
13. Child's agreement to be in a study.
14. ___ act of 1974.
15. Subjects whose identities are unknown are _____.

Down

2. Subjects should receive ___ ___ during a study.
3. Opposite of benefit; a factor that must be examined to determine whether a study is ethical.
5. Institutional Review Board.
8. Misinforming subjects.
9. Subject's permission to be in a study.
12. _____ are considered incompetent to give consent.

EXERCISES IN CRITIQUE

Directions: Review the research articles in Appendix B and answer the following questions.

1. Is the Sethares and Elliott (2004) study ethical? What information in the study indicates that the subjects' rights were protected and that institutional review was obtained?

2. Is the Wright (2003) study ethical? What information in the study indicates that the subjects' rights were protected and that institutional review was obtained?

3. Is the Zalon (2004) study ethical? What information in the study indicates that the subjects' rights were protected and that institutional review was obtained?

GOING BEYOND

Develop a proposal for a study. Discuss the benefit-risk ratio for conducting the study, develop a consent form, and complete an institutional review board (IRB) form for your study. Use the content in Chapter 9 to direct you in developing these aspects of a research proposal.

CHAPTER 10

Understanding Quantitative Research Design

INTRODUCTION

Read Chapter 10 and then complete the following exercises. These exercises will assist you in learning relevant terms and identifying and critiquing designs in published studies. The answers to these exercises are in Appendix A.

RELEVANT TERMS

Directions: Define the following terms in your own words without looking in your text. Then check your definitions with those in the glossary of your text. Using this strategy, you can identify elements of the term that are not yet clear in your mind. Reread the relevant section of the chapter to clarify your understanding of the term.

1. Analysis triangulation

2. Between method triangulation

3. Bias

4. Blocking

5. Carryover effect

6. Causality

7. Construct validity

8. Control group

9. Control

10. Counterbalancing

11. Covariation

12. Data triangulation

13. Design validity

14. Design

15. External validity

16. Extraneous variable

17. Fishing

18. Heterogeneity

19. History

20. Homogeneity

21. Intermediate mediation

22. Internal validity

23. Investigator triangulation

24. Manipulate

25. Manipulation

26. Matching

27. Maturation

28. Methodological triangulation

29. Micromediation

30. Molar

31. Monomethod bias

32. Mono-operation bias

33. Multicausality

34. Multiple triangulation

35. Necessary

36. Partial out

37. Probability

38. Randomized block design

39. Rival hypothesis

40. Selection

41. Statistical conclusion validity

42. Statistical regression

43. Stratification

44. Study validity

45. Sufficient

46. Theoretical triangulation

47. Threats to statistical conclusion validity

48. Threats to validity

49. Triangulation

50. Within method triangulation

KEY IDEAS
Directions: Fill in the blanks in the following sentences.

1. According to causality theory, things have causes, and causes lead to _____.

2. From the perspective of probability, a _____ may not produce a specific

    _____ each time that particular _____ occurs.

3. Designs are developed to reduce the possibilities and effects of _____.

4. The purpose of research designs is to maximize _____ of factors in the study situation.

5. The most commonly used manipulation in a study is the _____.

6. Critical analysis of research involves being able to think through

_____ that have occurred and make judgments about how seriously these affect the integrity of the findings.

7. Quasi-experimental and experimental studies are designed to examine

_____.

8. In most studies, _____ are the basis of obtaining valid answers.

9. Designs were developed to reduce threats to the validity of the _____.

MAKING CONNECTIONS
Directions: Match each term below with its definition or description.

Research Design Terms

a. Design validity
b. Multicausality
c. Descriptive design

d. Bias
e. Control
f. Internal validity

g. Probability
h. External validity
i. Correlational design

Definitions/Descriptions

_____   1. Deviates from the true or expected.
_____   2. The extent to which study findings can be generalized beyond the sample used in the study.
_____   3. The extent to which the effects detected in the study are a true reflection of reality.
_____   4. Addresses relative causality.
_____   5. Examines relationships between two or among more than two variables in a single group.
_____   6. The power to direct or manipulate factors to achieve a desired outcome.
_____   7. The study provides a convincing test of the framework propositions.
_____   8. The recognition that a number of interrelating variables can be involved in causing a particular effect.
_____   9. Gains more information about characteristics in a particular field of study.

Directions: Match the methods of design control listed below with the following statements describing the research design of a study. Note: Not all design control methods will be used.

Design Control Methods

a. Controlling the environment
b. Controlling subject and group equivalence
c. Control groups
d. Controlling the treatment
e. Counterbalancing

f. Controlling measurement
g. Controlling extraneous variables
h. Random sampling
i. Random assignment
j. Homogeneity

k. Heterogeneity
l. Blocking
m. Stratification
n. Matching
o. Statistical control

Statements

_____ 1. "Simple random sampling was used to select patients from the cardiac surgery operating room schedules over a 4-month period, yielding a sampling frame of approximately 800 patients" (Hanneman, 1994, p. 5).

_____ 2. "Chi-square demonstrated no significant differences between success and failure groups in gender, admitting diagnosis, type of surgery, cardiac rhythm, and weaning technique" (Hanneman, 1994, p. 5).

_____ 3. "Two successive heart rates had to be within five beats to ascertain that a steady state had been attained. If the fifth- and sixth-minute heart rates were not within five beats, the subject was asked to continue pedaling until a steady state was reached" (Neuberger, Kasal, Smith, Hassanein, & DeViney, 1994, p. 14).

_____ 4. "First, census block groups were selected using age, income, and ethnicity to facilitate the selection of a sample of menstruating women between the ages of 18 and 45 with a wide range of incomes. The ethnic mix was representative of the northwestern metropolitan area that was sampled" (Mitchell, Woods, & Lentz, 1994, p. 25).

_____ 5. "Criteria for inclusion were as follows: age between 18 and 45, not currently pregnant, not being treated for a gynecological problem, having menstrual periods, and the ability to write and understand English" (Mitchell, Woods, & Lentz, 1994, p.25).

_____ 6. "All interventions were tape recorded to control for content and order of presentation" (Melnyk, 1994, p. 50).

_____ 7. "Mothers listened to the appropriate audiotape in a private room, immediately following completion of demographic information and initial measures" (Melnyk, 1994, p. 50).

_____ 8. "To obtain sufficient power for analyses, data collection was designed to continue until at least 300 blue-collar, 200 skilled trades, and 100 white-collar subjects volunteered" (Lusk, Ronis, Kerr, & Atwood, 1994, p. 152)

_____ 9. "Data collectors alternated the order of mothers and fathers completing the instruments and doing the parent-infant interaction tasks. Different teaching tasks were alternately assigned to each parent" (Broom, 1994, p. 140).

_____ 10. "The research used a two-group independent sample experimental design. A randomized block design controlled for gender" (Treloar, 1994, p. 54).

PUZZLES

Word Scramble

Directions: Unscramble the sentence below by rearranging the letters to form actual words. Note: You will use all the letters in every word.

Sjut sa hte libunetpr rof a usheo tmus eb vidnuizliddaie ot eth fseccipi esuho giben itlub, os tsum eht anedig eb daem piseccif ot a yudst.

Secret Message

Directions: Translate the secret message below by substituting one letter for another. For example, if you decide that "c" should really be "x," then "c" will be "x" every time it appears in this puzzle. Hint: Try to translate short words first to establish vowel patterns.

Ymj uzwutxj tk f ijxnls nx yt xjy zu f xnyzfynts ymfy rfcnrnejx ymj utxxngnqnynjx

tk tgyfnsnsl fhhzwfyj fsxajwx yt tgojhynajx, vzjxyntsx, tw mdutymjxjx.

Crossword Puzzle

Directions: Complete the crossword puzzle on the next page. Note: If the answer is more than one word, there are no blank spaces left between the words.

Across

1. Selection of a control group subject who has similar characteristics to an experimental group subject.
4. Good design reduces threats to the validity of _____.
7. A cause leads to _____.
8. Administration of multiple treatments in random order.
10. The purpose of sampling criteria is to establish _____ among subjects.
12. Independent variable.

Down

2. A design strategy in which subjects with a wide variety of characteristics are obtained for the sample.
3. A visual depiction of the design.
5. To move around or control movement.
6. Group of subjects selected for a study.
8. Imposition of rules by the researcher to decrease the possibility of errors.
9. Controls the number of subjects at various levels of an extraneous variable in a sample.

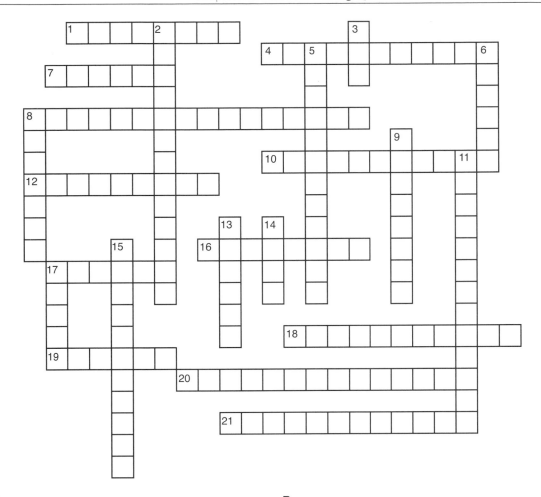

Across

16. An examination of whether the study provides a convincing test of the framework propositions.
17. A danger to the integrity of the findings.
18. Relative, rather than absolute, causality.
19. Blueprint for conducting a study.
20. Design strategy used to ensure even distribution of important variables throughout the sample.
21. Designs that provide greatest control in examining effects.

Down

11. Designs used to examine relationships between two or among more than two variables in a single group.
13. Strategy used to increase the probability of equivalence of sample to population.
14. Deviation of findings from the true.
15. Design used to provide a picture of situations as they naturally happen.
17. A design in which the patterns of responses of various samples are examined over time.

EXERCISES IN CRITIQUE

Directions: Review the research articles in Appendix B and answer the following questions.

1. Identify three sources of potential bias in the designs of the following studies.

    a.   Zalon's (2004) study

    b.   Sethares and Elliott's (2004) study

2. List three methods of control used in the designs of the following studies.

    a.   Zalon's (2004) study

    b.   Sethares and Elliott's (2004) study

3. To what populations can the findings from each of the following studies be generalized?

    a.   Zalon's (2004) study

    b.   Sethares and Elliott's (2004) study

4. What are the threats to external validity in each of the following studies?

   a. Zalon's (2004) study

   b. Sethares and Elliott's (2004) study

GOING BEYOND

Select a recently published study with a clearly stated framework. Examine the relationships among the study framework; the research objectives, questions, or hypotheses; and the design. Does the design allow an adequate test of the research objectives, questions, or hypotheses? Does the design facilitate application of the findings to the framework in the two quantitative studies presented in Appendix B?

CHAPTER 11

Selecting a Research Design

INTRODUCTION

Read Chapter 11 and then complete the following exercises. These exercises will assist you in understanding and selecting a design for a study. The answers to these exercises are in Appendix A.

RELEVANT TERMS

Directions: Define the following terms in your own words without looking in your text. Then check your definitions with those in the glossary of your text. Using this strategy, you can identify elements of the term that are not yet clear in your mind. Reread the relevant section of the chapter to clarify your understanding of the term.

1. Biased coin design

2. Carryover effect

3. Case study design

4. Classic experimental design

5. Clinical trial

6. Cohort

7. Comparative descriptive design

8. Comparative experimental design

9. Comparison group

10. Correlational study

11. Counterbalancing

12. Cross-sectional design

13. Crossover

14. Dependent variable

82

15. Descriptive design

16. Double-blinding

17. Early development trial

18. Endogenous variable

19. Event-partitioning design

20. Experimental design

21. Fatigue effect

22. Independent variable

23. Indicator

24. Inferred causality

25. Intervention

26. Late development effects

27. Longitudinal design

28. Matched pairs

29. Methodological design

30. Middle development trial

31. Model-testing design

32. Nested variables

33. One-group posttest-only design

34. One-group pretest-posttest design

35. Panel design

36. Phase I trial

37. Phase II trial

38. Phase III trial

39. Phase IV trial

40. Posttest only design with comparison group

41. Practice effect

42. Predictive design

43. Pre-experimental

44. Pretest sensitization

45. Primary prevention design

46. Prospective study

47. Quasi-experimental design

48. Random assignment to groups

49. Randomized block design

50. Randomized clinical trial

51. Residual variable

52. Retrospective study

53. SE trial

54. Secondary analysis design

55. Survey

56. Time dimensional design

57. Treatment

58. Treatment partitioning

59. Trend design

60. Truncated

61. Urn randomization

62. Washout period

KEY IDEAS

Directions: Fill in the blanks or provide the appropriate responses.

1. What is the purpose of a design?

2. Designs created to meet nursing needs need to be congruent with _____

   _____.

3. In epidemiological studies, _____ is an important dimension of the design.

4. Surveys are a means of gathering _____ data.

5. With a correlational design, it is important that the sample reflect:

6. The researcher cannot establish _____ using a correlational study.

7. In predictive correlational designs, independent variables most effective in prediction are

   _____ correlated with the dependent variable but _____ _____ correlated with other independent variables.

8. Interventions designed for use in quasi-experimental and experimental studies are expected to
   result in:

9. The power of a quasi-experimental or experimental design to examine causality is dependent
   on the degree to which:

10. The only acceptable way of maximizing the probability of equivalence between groups is

    _____ _____.

11. Variables found only at certain levels of the independent variable are called _____

_____ .

12. The research design organizes all the components of the study in a way that is most likely to lead to:

MAKING CONNECTIONS

Directions: Match the study designs listed below to the study descriptions that follow. Note: Some descriptions may match more than one design. Not all designs will be used.

Designs

a. Typical descriptive study
b. Comparative descriptive study
c. Longitudinal study
d. Trend study

e. Case study
f. Descriptive correlational study
g. Predictive correlational study

h. Model testing study
i. Quasi-experimental study
j. Experimental study

Study Descriptions

_____ 1. The purpose of the present study was to investigate the predictive relationships among attachment, selected demographic variables, and quality of life (Rickelman, Gallman, & Parra, 1994, p. 68).

_____ 2. The purpose of this study was to explore the dimensions of disturbing behaviors in institutionalized elders and to identify the related environmental and personal characteristics. A model comparison approach was used to examine the effectiveness of the Kaiser-Jones Model in explaining agitated psychomotor behavior (Kolanowski, Hurwitz, Taylor, Evans, & Strumpf, 1994, p. 73).

_____ 3. The purpose of this study was to determine whether men whose partners had experienced a low-risk pregnancy and men whose partners had been hospitalized during pregnancy for an obstetrical risk differed in paternal role competence from the time of their partners' early postpartum hospitalization to 1, 4, and 8 months after birth. Subjects were recruited during the 24th to 34th week of their partners' pregnancy and followed until 8 months after birth (Ferketich & Mercer, 1994, p. 82).

_____ 4. The purpose of this study was to describe health-promoting lifestyle behaviors among a sample of 187 African-American women (Ahijevych & Bernhard, 1994, p 86).

_____ 5. The purpose of this study was to evaluate an intervention given in prenatal classes during which prospective parents clarified their expectations. Couples participating in childbirth education classes at three private community hospitals were eligible for inclusion in the study. At a class session time selected by the instructor at each setting, the investigators conducted a 1-hour study session. Random assignment of experimental and control groups to each of the five prenatal instructors had been made previously (Coffman, Levitt, & Brown, 1994, p. 111).

_____ 6. The purpose of this study was to examine the effects of ovarian hormone cessation, hormone supplementation, and dietary fiber composition on body weight, appetite, and intestinal transit. In Part 1, effects of ovarian hormone status on body weight and baseline and stimulated intestinal transit were measured in chow-fed rats. Sprague-Dawley rats were ovariectomized (OVX), then injected daily (22 days) with estrogen (E), progesterone (P), the combination (E+P), or placebo. Controls were sham-operated and placebo-injected (Bond, Heitkemper, & Jarrett, 1994, p.18).

_____ 7. The purpose of the present study was to examine the relationship of two factors—self-efficacy and social support—to self-management in individuals with epilepsy (Dilorio, Faherty, & Manteuffel, 1992, p. 292).

Mapping the Design
Directions: Map the design for each of the following quasi-experimental studies.

1. "Transcutaneous oxygen and behavioral state data were collected before, during, and after a prescribed diagnostic heelstick. . . . The 5-minute period immediately preceding heelstick was the precry episode (baseline); the 5-minute period commencing with the heelstick was the cry episode; and the final 2-minute period was the postcry episode. . . . For the NNS infants, the pacifier was inserted immediately after heelstick. The ONNS infants did not receive the pacifier after heelstick and were allowed to cry without interference for the 5-minute crying episode" (Treloar, 1994, p. 52).

2. "All consenting patients admitted to the SICU had their admitting core temperature recorded. Patients with admitting core temperatures of less than 36°C were entered into the study. Their temperatures were recorded and shivering assessed every 15 minutes until they reached a core temperature of 36°C and remained at that temperature for 30 minutes. Patients were randomly assigned to one of three treatment groups (radiant heat, forced warm air, and warm blankets)" (Giuffre, Heidenreich, & Pruitt, 1994, p. 176).

EXERCISES IN CRITIQUE

Directions: Review the research articles in Appendix B and answer the following questions.

1. Identify the designs used in the following studies.

   a.   Zalon's (2004) study

   b.   Sethares and Elliott's (2004) study

2. What comparisons could be made given the designs used in the following studies?

   a.   Zalon's (2004) study

    b.   Sethares and Elliott's (2004) study

3. Identify three strengths in the designs used in each of the following studies.

    a.   Zalon's (2004) study

    b.   Sethares and Elliott's (2004) study

GOING BEYOND

Identify a quasi-experimental study in a recent nursing journal. Identify the intervention or treatment. Was the intervention described in sufficient detail for you to provide the same intervention? Was the intervention provided consistently to all subjects? In your opinion, was the intervention sufficiently powerful to cause a difference in effect between the experimental and control groups? Write a brief paragraph judging the adequacy of the intervention.

CHAPTER 12

Outcomes Research

INTRODUCTION

Read Chapter 12 and then complete the following exercises. These exercises will assist you in learning relevant terms and reading and comprehending published outcomes studies. The answers for these exercises are in Appendix A.

RELEVANT TERMS

Directions: Define the following terms in your own words without looking at your text. Then check your definitions with those in the glossary of your text. Using this strategy, you can identify elements of the term that are not yet clear in your mind. Reread the relevant section of the chapter to clarify your understanding of the term.

1. Aggregate

2. Clinical decision analysis

3. Consensus knowledge building

4. Cost-benefit analysis

5. Cost-effectiveness analysis

6. Donabedian's primordial cell

7. Efficiency

8. Geographic analysis

9. Health (as defined by Donabedian)

10. Individual

11. Interdisciplinary team

12. Intermediate end point

13. Latent transition analysis

14. Measurement error

15. Multicomponent treatments

16. Multilevel analysis

17. Numerical method

18. Opportunity costs

19. Out-of-pocket costs

20. Patient

21. Patient Outcomes Research Team (PORT) projects

22. Person

23. Population-based study

24. Practice pattern profiling

25. Prospective cohort study

26. Providers of care (as defined by Donabedian)

27. Research tradition

28. Retrospective cohort study

29. Sampling error

30. Small area analysis

31. Standard of care

32. Standardized mortality ratio

33. Structures of care

34. Subjects of care (as defined by Donabedian)

35. Treatment matching

36. Variance analysis

KEY IDEAS

Directions: Fill in the blanks or provide the appropriate responses.

1. Outcomes research focuses on:

2. The meeting of which two National Institutes of Health study sections ultimately led to the development of the Agency for Health Services Research (AHSR)?

   a.

   b.

3. What was the first large-scale study to examine factors influencing patient outcomes?

4. The Medical Outcomes Study (MOS) was flawed because it failed to control for the following three elements:

   a.

   b.

   c.

5. The following three components, commonly performed by nurses, were considered by MOS to be components of medical practice:

   a.

   b.

   c.

6. Identify three questions that might be addressed by PORTs.

   a.

   b.

   c.

7. Clinical guideline panels were developed to:

8. Examining the impact of nursing on overall hospital outcomes will require:

9. To evaluate an outcome, the outcome must be _____ to the

   _____ that _____ the outcome.

10. In outcomes research, the _____ must clarify what outcomes are
    desirable.

11. List three examples of standards of care.

    a.

    b.

    c.

12. _____ samples are preferred in outcome studies.

13. To allow evaluation or monitoring of individual patient care, the following information must be
    available in large databases:

    a.

    b.

    c.

    d.

14. Decision analysis is based on the following four assumptions:

    a.

    b.

    c.

    d.

15. From an outcomes research perspective, three questions that might be asked about interventions
    are:

    a.

b.

c.

16. Treatment matching is used when the following conditions are met:

    a.

    b.

    c.

17. Outcomes selected for nursing studies should be those that are

    _____.

18. Instruments for outcomes studies should be selected for their sensitivity to

    _____.

19. The Nursing Care Report Card for Acute Care was developed by

    _____.

20. List five fallacies identified by Gottman and Rushe (1993) held by researchers related to the analysis of change.

    a.

    b.

    c.

    d.

    e.

21. In analyzing improvement of patients' treatment with a particular intervention, the following parameters should be reported:

    a.

    b.

    c.

    d.

22. In performing variance analysis, it is important to track:

    a.

    b.

    c.

Making Connections

Directions: Match the researchers with their contributions to outcomes research.

Researchers

a. Louis
b. Hinshaw
c. Wennberg
d. Donabedian
e. Sir William Petty

f. Chaput de Saintonge and colleagues
g. Lange and Jacox
h. Earnest A. Codman
i. Maynard

j. Florence Nightingale
k. Schmitt, Farrell, and Heinemann
l. Semmelweiss
m. Kelly and colleagues

Research Contributions

_____ 1. Proposed a method evaluating the effectiveness of care based on an examination of the patient 1 year after surgery or discharge from a hospital.

_____ 2. The first physician to question the effectiveness of medical care.

_____ 3. One of the first nurses to conduct outcome studies.

_____ 4. Examined small area variations in medical practice.

_____ 5. As director of the National Institute for Nursing Research, sponsored the Conference on Patient Outcomes Research: Examining the Effectiveness of Nursing Practice.

_____ 6. Viennese physician who used hospital records to show that women in labor who were assisted by midwives had lower mortality rates than those attended by physicians in hospital wards.

_____ 7. Criticized the MOS for not considering the influence of nursing actions while studying medical practice outcomes.

_____ 8. Recommended elements necessary to the description of interventions.

_____ 9. Developed a strategy for analyzing clinical decisions using "paper patients."

_____ 10. The first to use statistical methods to examine the effectiveness of medical interventions.

_____ 11. Proposed a theory of quality health care and the process of evaluating it.

_____ 12. Identified important health policy questions related to nursing that should be examined using large databases.

_____ 13. Identified the characteristics of interdisciplinary teams.

PUZZLES

Word Scramble

Directions: Unscramble the sentence below by rearranging the letters to form actual words. Note: You will use all the letters in every word.

Het tomrnenum rollpengip scemouto sharcere si mongic morf ployci karnrse, rinsures, dan eht plibuc.

Secret Message

Directions: Translate the secret message below by substituting one letter for another. For example, if you decide that "c" should really be "x," then "c" will be "x" every time it appears in this puzzle. Hint: Try to translate short words first to establish vowel patterns.

Csy wcpxcynzyw kwyr zo jkcmjiy pywyxpms xpy, cj wniy ydcyoy, x rybxpcqpy

gpji csy xmmybcyr wmzyoczgzm iycsjr.

Crossword Puzzle

Directions: Complete the crossword puzzle on the next page. Note: If the answer is more than one word, there are no blank spaces left between the words.

Across

1. A norm on which quality of care is judged.
4. _____ _____ analysis—technique used to determine alternate ways of using resources to produce the greatest net benefit.
6. Someone who has already gained access to care.
8. Someone who may or may not have gained access to care.
11. A group of people identified at a point of time as being at risk for or experiencing a health condition.

Down

2. Those expenses incurred by the patient or family that are not reimbursable by the insurance company.
3. Difference between what exists in reality and what is measured.
5. Elements of organization and administration that guide the processes of care.
7. _____ analysis—Used to examine variations in patterns of care by geographic area.
9. Proximate outcomes.

Across

16. Very early statistical procedures developed by Louis.
20. _____ (economic)—the least costly method of achieving a desired end with the maximum benefit to be obtained from available resources.
21. _____ analysis—used to track individual and group variance from a specific critical pathway.

Down

10. Individual practitioners, who might be of the same profession or different professions, working concurrently, as individuals, or as a team.
12. Lost prospects that the patient, family member, or others experience as a consequence of illness.

Across

22. Single person or patient.
23. Defines acceptable research methodologies for a particular research focus.

Down

13. The difference between a sample statistic used to estimate a population parameter and the actual but unknown value.
14. A patient, a person, a caseload, a community.
15. The physical-physiologic function of the individual patient being cared for by the individual practitioner.
17. _____ analysis—studies how environmental factors, individual attributes, and behavior interact to influence health.
18. A case load, target population, or community.
19. _____ _____ analysis—examination of patterns of use by geographical area.

GOING BEYOND

Identify nursing outcome studies published in the last 12 months. Evaluate the methodology of the studies for the purposes of outcome research. How do these studies contribute to nursing needs for knowledge related to patient outcomes?

CHAPTER 13

Intervention Research

INTRODUCTION

Read Chapter 13 and then complete the following exercises. These exercises will assist you in understanding and selecting a design for a study. The answers to these exercises are in Appendix A.

RELEVANT TERMS

Directions: Define the following terms in your own words without looking in your text. Then check your definitions with those in the glossary of your text. Using this strategy, you can identify elements of the term that are not yet clear in your mind. Reread the relevant section of the chapter to clarify your understanding of the term.

1. Adaptation

2. Advanced testing

3. Analogue situation

4. Causal connection

5. Causal dynamics

6. Causal explanation

7. Clinical guideline

8. Complex interventions

9. Complexity

10. Confounding variable

11. Constructive strategy

12. Creating a demand

13. Critical pathway

14. Descriptive theory

15. Disadvantaged group

16. Dismantling strategy (substruction design)

17. Duration

18. Extraneous factors

19. Factorial ANOVA designs

20. Field test

21. Formal test

22. Fractional factorial designs

23. Integrity of intervention

24. Intensity

25. Intermediate outcomes

26. Intervener

27. Intervention

28. Intervention complexity

29. Intervention dose

30. Intervention duration

31. Intervention effectiveness

32. Intervention integrity

33. Intervention intensity

34. Intervention research

35. Intervention strength

36. Intervention taxonomy

37. Intervention theory

38. Key informant

39. Lack of intervention integrity

40. Logical-positivist

41. Mediating process

42. Mediator variable

43. Modeling the intervention

44. Moderator variable

45. Natural leader

46. Nursing intervention

47. Observation system

48. Participatory research

49. Participatory research strategy

50. Pilot test

51. Potential market

52. Preference clinical trial

53. Prescriptive theory

54. Product sampling

55. Project team

56. Prototype

57. Reinvention

58. Response surface

59. Response surface methodology

60. Sampling

61. Stakeholder

62. Strength

63. Structural equation analysis

64. Technical support

65. Timing

66. Treatment matching

67. True experiment

68. Type II error

69. Type III error

70. Use standards

71. Validity of the cause

KEY IDEAS

Directions: Fill in the blanks or provide the appropriate responses.

1. Intervention research in nursing holds great promise for

   _____.

2. The _____ is being seriously questioned by a growing number of schol-
   ars because modifications in the original design have decreased its validity.

3. A nursing intervention can be defined in what four ways?

   a.

   b.

   c.

   d.

4. In medical and nursing research, the "true experiment" is commonly referred to as a

   _____.

5. In causal explanation, required in intervention theory research, in addition to demonstrating that the intervention causes the outcome, the researcher must provide scientific evidence to

   _____

   _____.

6. A participatory research strategy involves including representatives from

   _____ as collaborators.

7. An intervention theory includes a descriptive theory, which describes the causal processes, and a prescriptive theory, which specifies what must be done to achieve the desired results. The prescriptive theory includes:

   a.

   b.

   c.

8. Strength of the intervention is defined in terms of the _____,

   _____, and _____.

9. A moderator is a separate _____ variable affecting outcomes.

10. Extraneous variables, sometimes referred to as _____ _____, are elements of the environment or characteristics of the patient that significantly affect the problem, the treatment process, or the outcomes.

MAKING CONNECTIONS
Directions: Match each term below with its appropriate description.

Designing an Intervention

a. Pilot testing
b. Analogue testing
c. Testing variations in effectiveness

d. Formal testing
e. Developing a prototype
f. Treatment matching
g. Field test

h. Preference clinical trial
i. Path analysis
j. Component testing

Descriptions

_____   1. A primitive design.

_____   2. Using actors to play roles in the intervention.

_____   3. Small studies to determine whether the prototype will work.

_____   4. Rigorous test of the intervention.

_____   5. Advanced testing.

_____   6. Examination of causal processes through which every component of the intervention has its effect.

_____   7. Testing the effective of active choice of subjects for intervention on outcomes.

_____   8. Comparison of relative effectiveness of various treatments.

_____   9. Testing differential effects of complex interventions.

_____   10. Testing intervention in uncontrolled clinical setting.

PUZZLES

Word Scramble

Directions: Unscramble the sentence below by rearranging the letters to form actual words. Note: You will use all the letters in every word.

Revittenspinon stum eb seddirebe roem lordaby sa lal fo het catoisn quireder ot sadreds a cultrapira moplemb.

Secret Message

Directions: Translate the secret message below by substituting one letter for another. For example, if you decide that "g" should really be "f," then "g" will be "f" every time it appears in this puzzle. Hint: Try to translate short words first to establish vowel patterns.

Sehuh dt jruuhysan adssah jxytdtshyjn dy seh whugxuzlyjh xg ly

dyshuqhysdxy.

Crossword Puzzle

Directions: Complete the crossword puzzle below. Note: If the answer is more than one word, there are no blank spaces left between the words.

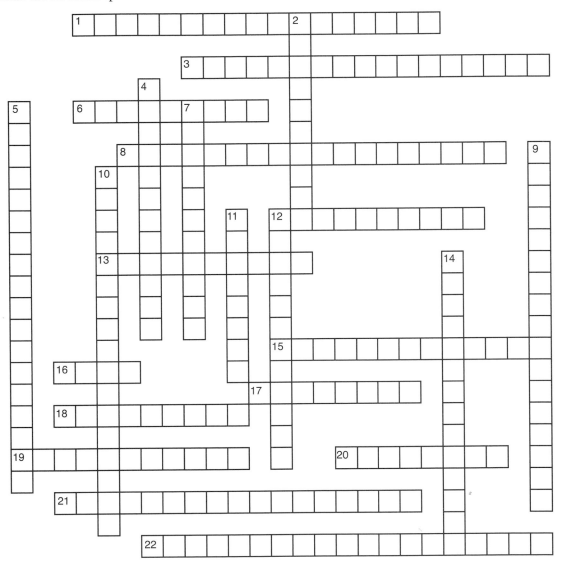

Across

1. Performed to compare the relative effectiveness of various treatments.
3. Occurs with the intervention and alters the causal relationship between the intervention and outcomes.
6. Force, power, or amount of an intervention.
8. Minorities, the poor, the elderly, etc.
12. The person providing the intervention.
13. Level of difficulty in understanding or using.
15. _____ (intervention)—extent to which treatment is successful.
16. _____ (intervention)—amount of the intervention at a specific point in time.
17. Potency of the intervention.
18. _____ (of intervention)—intervention administered exactly as directed.
19. Changing the intervention to fit existing conditions.
20. Length of time the treatment must be provided.
21. Allows researchers to observe events related to the intervention naturalistically.
22. Occurs prior to the final result.

Down

2. Modification to meet the agency's need.
4. Important provider of information.
5. Prescribes actions to be taken by caregivers in a given situation.
7. A person or group who will be affected by a change.
9. Variables external to the phenomenon described.
10. A researcher who adheres to an atheoretical research strategy that focuses on discovering laws through the accumulation of facts.
11. _____ (intervention)—categorization of interventions.
12. Deliberative activity directed toward accomplishing particular therapeutic objectives.
14. Requires rigid adherence to design rules, including random sampling, equivalence of groups, complete control of the treatment, a control group that receives no treatment, control of the environment, and precise measurement of variables.

EXERCISES IN CRITIQUE

Directions: Review the intervention described in Sethares and Elliott's (2004) study in Appendix B and answer the following questions.

1. Is the intervention described in sufficient detail for you to provide the intervention?

2. Is the intervention theory-based?

GOING BEYOND

1. If you were to use Sethares & Elliott's intervention for a research program following intervention theory strategies, how would you plan the program of research?

2. Search the nursing literature for a nursing study using intervention theory methodology. Identify the process used to develop the intervention. Describe the method of observation used during the process. Was the intervention theory clearly presented? Was the intervention described in sufficient detail for you to provide the same intervention? Was the intervention provided consistently to all subjects? In your opinion, was the intervention sufficiently powerful to cause a difference in effect between the experimental and control groups? Write a brief paragraph judging the adequacy of the intervention.

CHAPTER 14

Sampling

INTRODUCTION

Read Chapter 14 and then complete the following exercises. These exercises will assist you in understanding the sampling process in published studies. The answers to these exercises are in Appendix A.

RELEVANT TERMS

Directions: Match each term below with its correct definition.

Terms

a. Accessible population
b. Cluster sampling
c. Convenience sampling
d. Network sampling
e. Nonprobability sampling

f. Probability sampling
g. Purposive sampling
h. Quote sampling
i. Random sampling
j. Sampling

k. Sample criteria
l. Stratified random sampling
m. Systematic sampling
n. Target population
o. Theoretical sampling

Definitions

_____ 1. Process of selecting a group of people, events, behaviors, or other elements that are representative of the population being studied.

_____ 2. Portion of the target population to which the researcher has reasonable access.

_____ 3. All elements (individuals, objects, events, or substances) that meet the sample criteria for inclusion in a study.

_____ 4. Judgmental sampling that involves the conscious selection by the researcher of certain subjects or elements to include in a study.

_____ 5. List of the characteristics essential for membership in the target population.

_____ 6. Random sampling technique in which every member (element) of the population has a probability higher than zero of being selected for the sample; examples include simple random sampling, stratified random sampling, cluster sampling, and systematic sampling.

_____ 7. Sampling technique selecting every kth individual from an ordered list of all members of a population, using a random selected starting point.

_____ 8. Random selection of elements from the sampling frame for inclusion in a study.

_____ 9. Sampling technique used when the researcher knows some of the variables in the population that are critical to achieving representativeness; the sample is divided into strata or groups using these identified variables.

_____ 10. Sampling technique in which a frame is developed that includes a list of all states, cities, institutions, or organizations (clusters) that could be used in a study; a randomized sample is drawn from this list.

_____ 11. "Snowballing" technique that takes advantage of social networks and the fact that friends tend to hold characteristics in common; subjects meeting sample criteria are asked to assist in locating others with similar characteristics.

_____ 12. Sampling in which not every element of the population has an opportunity for selection, such as convenience sampling, quota sampling, purposive sampling, and network sampling.

_____ 13. Convenience sampling technique with an added strategy to ensure the inclusion of subjects who are likely to be underrepresented in the convenience sample, such as women, minority groups, and uneducated persons.

_____ 14. Sampling technique that involves including subjects in a study because they happen to be in the right place at the right time.

_____ 15. Sampling method often used in grounded theory research to advance the development of a theory throughout the research process. The researcher gathers data from any individual or group that can provide relevant data for theory generation.

KEY IDEAS
Directions: Fill in the blanks or provide the appropriate responses.

1. The individual units of a population are called _____, and if these units are people,

they are called _____.

2. The researcher desires to obtain a sample from an accessible population and generalize to a

_____ _____.

3. Representativeness means that the _____, _____ _____,

and _____ _____ are alike in as many ways as possible.

4. Identify two ways you might evaluate the representativeness of a sample in a published study.

a.

b.

5. Random variation is:

6. A list of every member of a population is referred to as a _____

_____.

7. A sampling plan outlines the:

8. In critiquing the sampling plan in a study, several things are examined. List at least three things you need to examine.

a.

b.

c.

9. When the sampling criteria are narrowly defined or very specific, the sample desired is

_____.

10. When the sampling criteria are broadly defined to include a variety of subjects, the sample

desired is _____.

11. Subjects must be over the age of 18, able to read and write English, newly diagnosed with

cancer, and have no other major illnesses. These are examples of _____

_____.

12. The sample was 65% female and 40% African-American, 30% Hispanic, and 30% Caucasian.

These are examples of _____ _____.

13. When subjects die or withdraw from the study, this is referred to as _____

_____.

14. The term control group is limited to only those studies using _____ sampling methods.

15. If _____ sampling methods are used for sample selection, the group not receiving the treatment is referred to as a comparison group.

16. Identify four types of probability sampling.

    a.

    b.

    c.

    d.

17. If the original group of subjects is selected randomly prior to random assignment to treatment or control groups, it is considered a _____ sample.

18. Identify four types of nonprobability sampling.

    a.

    b.

    c.

    d.

19. Currently, the majority of nursing studies use _____ (*probability* or *nonprobability*) sampling methods.

20. Convenience sampling is also called _____ _____.

21. Purposive sampling is referred to as _____ _____.

22. The adequacy of the sample size can be evaluated using _____ _____.

23. Power is the capacity to detect _____ or _____ that actually exist in the population.

24. The minimal acceptable level of power for a study is _____.

25. If the findings of a study are nonsignificant, the researcher should examine the adequacy of the sample size by running a _____ _____.

26. Effect size is the extent to which the _____ _____ is false.

27. Identify five factors that influence the adequacy of a quantitative study's sample size.

    a.

    b.

    c.

    d

    e.

28. Identify three sampling methods that are commonly used in qualitative research.

    a.

    b.

    b.

29. A qualitative study that included subjects selected based on their history of substance abuse and their judged severity of abuse over the last year used _____ sampling method.

30. List four factors that need to be considered in determining the sample size of a qualitative study.

    a.

    b.

    c.

    d.

31. Identify the types of research settings used in nursing studies.

    a.

    b.

    c.

32. _____ setting is an uncontrolled, real-life situation or environment for the conduct of a study.

33. _____ _____ setting is an artificially constructed environment for the sole purpose of doing research.

34. _____ _____ setting is an environment that is manipulated or modified in some way by the researcher but usually in a limited way.

35. The two types of sampling criteria that might be used in a study are _____ and

_____ criteria.

MAKING CONNECTIONS

Directions: Match the sampling methods listed below with the examples of sampling methods from published studies. Note: Some sampling methods will be used more than once.

Sampling Methods

a. Cluster sampling
b. Convenience sampling
c. Network sampling

d. Purposive sampling
e. Quota sampling
f. Simple random sampling

g. Stratified random sampling
h. Systematic sampling
i. Theoretical sampling

Examples

_____ 1. Five hundred nurses were randomly selected from a list of all registered nurses in the state of Texas.

_____ 2. A sample of 50 patients with diabetes was obtained from patients who came to an outpatient clinic; those 50 patients were randomly placed in the comparison and experimental groups.

_____ 3. A sample of 10 HIV-positive subjects was obtained by asking 3 subjects to identify friends with HIV who might participate in the study.

_____ 4. A sample of 1,000 critical care nurses was obtained by asking 100 critical care nurse managers in 50 randomly selected, large hospitals to identify 10 staff nurses to complete a survey.

_____ 5. Subjects with a history of having asthma were recruited to provide relevant information to develop a theory of asthma management.

_____ 6. Gender was used to stratify a sample of 100 randomly selected subjects.

_____ 7. The researcher obtained a list of all certified nurse practitioners, picked a random starting point, and then selected every twenty-fifth individual to participate in the study.

_____ 8. Fifty hypertensive subjects were recruited in a clinic to participate in a study.

_____ 9. An equal number of patients with asthma, emphysema, and chronic bronchitis were recruited from the local Better Breathers chapter to participate in a study.

_____ 10. The sample included 50 patients; 25 were examples of strong self-care, and 25 were examples of poor self-care.

_____ 11. Five thousand military personnel were randomly selected to participate in a study.

_____ 12. A sample of drug-addicted nurses was obtained by asking five subjects to identify friends who were drug-addicted.

_____ 13. Twenty-five home health patients were asked to participate in a study because they had a history of pressure ulcers that would not heal.

_____ 14. Ten subjects were selected because they could provide relevant data for the generation of a theory of pain management and assessment.

_____ 15. Fifty surgery patients were randomly selected from a hospital and randomly placed in control and treatment groups.

Directions: Match the types of settings listed below with the examples of settings from published studies. Note: Some types of settings will be used more than once.

Types of Settings

a. Highly controlled setting
b. Natural setting
c. Partially controlled setting

Examples

_____ 1. Research unit in a pediatric hospital

_____ 2. Home of a patient who is on continuous oxygen

_____ 3. School for severely disabled children

_____ 4. A rehabilitation center that has a structured protocol for exercise activities

_____ 5. Rat research on new drugs done in a pharmaceutical lab

PUZZLES

Crossword Puzzle

Directions: Complete the crossword puzzle below. Note: If the answer is more than one word, there are no blank spaces left between the words.

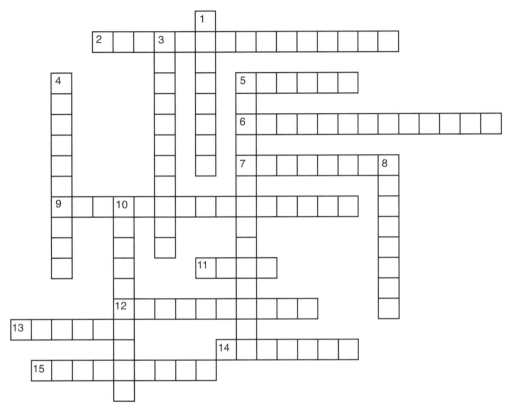

Across

2. Group in a study.
5. Equal opportunity to be a subject.
6. Used to determine sample size.
7. _____ make up the population.
9. Used to select subjects.
11. Slanted from truth.
12. Portion of the target population within the range of researcher.
13. Population designated by sample criteria.
14. Possible sampling method used when studying subjects with HIV.
15. Nonprobability sampling method.

Down

1. _____ determine who is in a sample.
3. Random sampling.
4. Number of subjects in a study.
5. Sample is _____ of population.
8. People in a study.
10. All members of a refined set of elements.

EXERCISES IN CRITIQUE

Sethares and Elliott Study

Directions: Review the Sethares and Elliott (2004) research article in Appendix B and answer the following questions.

1. Identify the study population.

2. List the sample criteria for this study.

3. Identify the sample characteristics for this study.

4. What is the sample size? Was a power analysis used to determine the sample size?

5. Was the sample size adequate? Provide a rationale.

6. What was the sample mortality for this study?

7. Was probability or nonprobability sampling used in this study? What specific type of sampling method was used in this study?

8. Was the sample in this study representative of the target population? Provide a rationale.

9. Can the findings be generalized? Provide a rationale.

Wright Study

Directions: Review the Wright (2003) research article in Appendix B and answer the following questions.

1. Identify the study population.

2. List the sample criteria for this study.

3. Identify the sample characteristics for this study.

4. What is the sample size? Was a power analysis used to determine the sample size?

5. Was the sample size adequate? Provide a rationale.

6. What was the sample mortality for this study?

7. Was probability or nonprobability sampling used in this study? What specific type of sampling method was used in this study?

8. Was the sample in this study representative of the population studied? Provide a rationale.

9. Can the findings be generalized? Provide a rationale.

Zalon Study

Directions: Review the Zalon (2004) research article in Appendix B and answer the following questions.

1. Identify the study population.

2. List the sample criteria for this study.

3. Identify the sample characteristics for this study.

4. What is the sample size? Was a power analysis used to determine the sample size?

5. Was the sample size adequate? Provide a rationale.

6. What was the sample mortality for this study?

7. Was probability or nonprobability sampling used in this study? What specific type of sampling method was used in this study?

8. Was the sample in this study representative of the population studied? Provide a rationale.

9. Can the findings be generalized? Provide a rationale.

STUDY SETTINGS

Directions: Identify the type of setting for each of the studies in Appendix B. Note: More than one type of setting may apply to each study.

Setting Types

a. Natural setting
b. Partially controlled setting
c. Highly controlled setting

Studies

_____   1. Sethares and Elliott (2004)
_____   2. Wright (2003)
_____   3. Zalon (2004)

CHAPTER 15

The Concepts of Measurement

INTRODUCTION

Read Chapter 15 and then complete the following exercises. These exercises will assist you in learning relevant terms and evaluating measures in relation to concepts important to measurement. The answers to these exercises are in Appendix A.

RELEVANT TERMS

Directions: Define the following terms in your own words without looking at your text. Then check your definitions with those in the glossary of your text. Using this strategy, you can identify elements of the term that are not yet clear in your mind. Reread the relevant section of the chapter to clarify your understanding of the term.

1. Absolute zero point

2. Accuracy

3. Alternate forms reliability

4. Concurrent validity

5. Construct domain

6. Construct universe

7. Construct validity

8. Content-related validity evidence

9. Contrasting groups validity

10. Convergent validity

11. Criterion-referenced testing

12. Direct measurement

13. Discriminate analysis validity

121

14. Divergent validity

15. Equivalence

16. Error in physiologic measures

17. Error score

18. Extreme cases

19. Face validity

20. Freedom from drift

21. Frequency response

22. Fundamentalist

23. Holistic fallacy

24. Homogeneity

25. Indirect measurement

26. Instrumentation

27. Internal consistency

28. Interpretive reliability

29. Interrater reliability

30. Interval-scale measurement

31. Levels of measurement

32. Measurement

33. Measurement error

34. Metric ordinal scale

35. Multimethod-multitrait method

36. Nominal-scale measurement

37. Norm-referenced testing

38. Observed score

39. Ordered metric scale

40. Ordinal-scale measurement

41. Outliers

42. Parallel forms reliability

43. Physiological measures

44. Pragmatists

45. Precision

46. Predictive validity

47. Random error

48. Ratio-scale measurement

49. Readability

50. Referencing

KEY IDEAS

Directions: Fill in the blanks or provide the appropriate responses.

1. The purpose of measurement is to produce _____ data.

2. The ideal, perfect measure is referred to as the _____ measure.

3. Measurement _____ is the difference between true measure and what, in reality, is measured.

4. Weight is an example of _____ measurement.

5. A coping scale is an example of _____ measurement.

6. A reliability value of _____ is considered the lowest acceptable coefficient for a well-developed measurement tool.

7. Describe three situations that might result in random error.

   a.

   b.

   c.

8. Describe three measurement situations that might result in systematic error.

   a.

   b.

   c.

MAKING CONNECTIONS

Directions: Identify the type of measurement error likely to occur with each of the measurement methods.

Error Types

a. Random error
b. Systematic error

Measurement Methods

_____   1. Community income using a white, middle-class sample
_____   2. Severity of cancer at diagnosis in community, using patients in a county hospital
_____   3. Average body weight measured at work at noon
_____   4. Blood pressure taken with a stethoscope with which it is difficult to hear
_____   5. Scores on drug calculation test taken in clinical setting anytime during work shift

Directions: Match the measurement levels listed below with the specific types of measures that follow.

Measurement Levels

a. Nominal
b. Ordinal
c. Interval or higher

Types of Measures

_____   1.   Temperature

_____   2.   Gender

_____   3.   Educational level

_____   4.   Final exam grade

_____   5.   Type of cancer

_____   6.   Severity of illness rank

_____   7.   Score from visual analogue scale

Directions: Match each reliability or validity type with its definition.

Reliability or Validity Types

a. Test-retest reliability
b. Interrater reliability
c. Homogeneity
d. Content validity
e. Validity evidence from contrasting groups

f. Validity evidence from examining convergence
g. Validity evidence from examining divergence
h. Validity evidence from discriminant analysis

i. Validity evidence from predicting future events
j. Validity evidence from predicting concurrent events
k. Accuracy
l. Precision
m. Sensitivity

Definitions

_____   1.   Comparison of values with those of other instruments that measure the same concept

_____   2.   Amount of change that can be measured

_____   3.   Comparison of values with those of other instruments that measure similar concepts

_____   4.   Consistency of measurement of two raters

_____   5.   Comparison of groups expected to have opposing responses to instrument items

_____   6.   Adequacy of operational definition

_____   7.   Evaluates consistency of repeated measures

_____   8.   Comparison of values with those of other instruments that measure opposite concepts

_____ 9. Ability of instrument values to predict future performance

_____ 10. Ability to predict current value of measure based on value from measure of another concept

_____ 11. Correlation of various items within an instrument

_____ 12. Consistency of measurement

_____ 13. Extent to which all elements of a concept are measured

PUZZLES

Word Scramble

Directions: Unscramble the sentence below by rearranging the letters to form actual words. Note: You will use all the letters in every word.

Rethe si on fertpec semarue.

Secret Message

Directions: Translate the secret message below by substituting one letter for another. For example, if you decide that "y" should really be "p," then "y" will be "p" every time it appears in this puzzle. Hint: Try to translate short words first to establish vowel patterns.

Anurjkrurch cnbcrwp wnnmd cx kn ynaoxavnm xw njlq rwbcadvnwc dbnm rw j

bcdmh.

Crossword Puzzle

Directions: Complete the crossword puzzle below. Note: If the answer is more than one word, there are no blank spaces left between the words.

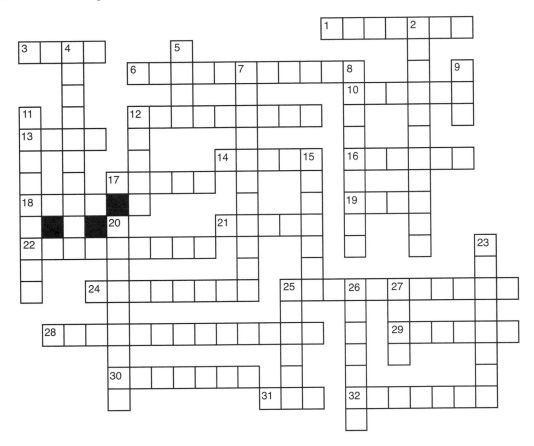

Across

1. Gather data.
3. Most common method of obtaining questionnaire data.
6. Strategies used to produce trustworthy data.
10. The crudest form of scale.
12. Concerned with the consistency of repeated measures.
13. Infrequent occurrence.
14. Highest level of measurement.
16. Self-report measures with summated scores.
17. The difference between true measure and what is measured.

Down

2. Interrater reliability.
4. Measurement method.
5. Information obtained through measurement.
7. Consistency of measurement.
8. Score obtained if no measurement error.
9. Commonly used demographic data.
11. Reproducibility of measurements.
12. A measurement tool can be used to generate a _____ for each subject for a study variable.
15. Subjective form of measurement used commonly in qualitative research.

Across

18. Thought related to a creative way to measure a nursing phenomenon.
19. Unstructured.
21. Site of data collection.
22. Measurement strategy involving verbal communication between the researcher and the subject.
24. Evaluation of the adequacy of a physiologic operational definition.
25. The amount of change of a parameter that can be measured precisely.
28. A printed self-report form with individual items that are not summated.
29. Scale with options rated from negative to positive.
30. Level of measurement in which values must be ranked.
31. Common method of obtaining demographic data.
32. Lowest level of measurement.

Down

20. Approach to judging reliability of physiologic measures.
23. Level of measurement with equal numerical distances.
25. Selye identified and measured the concept of _____ in his research.
26. Place in which data collection occurs.
27. Common source of interview data.

EXERCISES IN CRITIQUE

Directions: Review the Zalon (2004) and Sethares and Elliott (2004) studies in Appendix B and answer the following questions.

1. Using the following tables, identify the variables measured, the method of measurement, and the directness of measurement (D = direct, I = indirect).

Zalon Study

Variable	Method of Measurement	Directness

Sethares and Elliott Study

Variable	Method of Measurement	Directness

2. Now examine the reliability and validity of each measure in the two studies. For each table below, first identify the measure. Then, within the table, identify the types of reliability and validity reported for each measure and the numerical values reported for each. Of particular interest is whether reliability was examined in the sample used.

Zalon Study

a. Measure _____

Type of Reliability and Validity	Value	From present sample?

b. Measure _____

Type of Reliability or Validity	Value	From present sample?

c. Measure _____

Type of Reliability or Validity	Value	From present sample?

d. Measure _____

Type of Reliability or Validity	Value	From present sample?

e. Measure _____

Type of Reliability or Validity	Value	From present sample?

Sethares and Elliott Study

a. Measure _____

Type of Reliability or Validity	Value	From present sample?

b. Measure _____

Type of Reliability or Validity	Value	From present sample?

c. Measure _____

Type of Reliability or Validity	Value	From present sample?

3. Using the information gathered above, judge the adequacy of the measurement methods used in each study.

   a.   Zalon study

   b.   Sethares and Elliott study

CHAPTER 16

Measurement Strategies in Nursing

INTRODUCTION

Read Chapter 16 and then complete the following exercises. These exercises will assist you in learning relevant terms and identifying and critiquing measurement procedures in published studies. The answers to these exercises are in Appendix A.

RELEVANT TERMS

Directions: Define the following terms in your own words without looking at your text. Then check your definitions with those in the glossary of your text. Using this strategy, you can identify elements of the term that are not yet clear in your mind. Reread the relevant section of the chapter to clarify your understanding of the term.

1. Checklist

2. Delphi technique

3. Diaries

4. Direct measurement

5. Forced choice

6. Indirect measurement

7. Interviews

8. Likert scales

9. Magnitude scaling

10. Observational measurement

11. Physiological measurement

12. Probing

13. Projective techniques

14. Q methodology

15. Questionnaires

16. Rating scales

17. Response set

18. Scales

19. Self-report

20. Semantic differentials

21. Structured interviews

22. Structured observation

23. Visual analogue scales

KEY IDEAS

Directions: Fill in the blanks or provide the appropriate responses.

1. Knowledge of measurement methods in nursing is important at _____ levels of nursing.

2. For some measures, such as dizziness, _____ may be the only means of obtaining information needed for research.

3. _____ physiologic measures are most valid.

4. One disadvantage of using sensors to measure physiologic variables is that the presence of a transducer within the body can:

5. In observational measurement, as with any type of measurement, _____ is very important.

6. Structured interviews include strategies that provide increasing amounts of _____

   by the researcher over the _____ of the interview.

7. There is a _____ response rate to interviews than to questionnaires.

8. Compared with interviews, questionnaires tend to have less _____.

9. Scales are a more _____ means of measuring phenomena than are questionnaires.

10. What is the most commonly used scaling technique?

11. What type of scale has the finest discrimination of values?

12. What is the name (and common abbreviated name) of the computerized database for locating existing measurement methods?

MAKING CONNECTIONS
Directions: Match each measurement method with its description.

Measurement Methods

a. Physiologic measures
b. Unstructured observation
c. Structured observation
d. Unstructured interview
e. Structured interview

f. Questionnaire
g. Rating scale
h. Likert scale
i. Semantic differential
j. Q methodology

k. Visual analogue scale
l. Delphi technique
m. Projective technique
n. Diary

Descriptions

_____ 1. Involves spontaneously observing and recording what is seen

_____ 2. A printed self-report form in which subjects provide written responses to closed-ended questions

_____ 3. A record of events kept by the subject

_____ 4. Usually norm-referenced

_____ 5. Magnitude scaling

_____ 6. A technique of comparative rating that preserves the subjective point of view of the individual

_____ 7. The crudest form of scaling technique

_____ 8. Based on the assumption that the responses of individuals to unstructured or ambiguous situations reflect the attitudes, desires, personality characteristics, and motives of the individual

_____ 9. Designed to determine the opinion or attitude of a subject and contains a number of declarative statements with a scale after each statement

_____ 10. Consists of two opposite adjectives with a seven-point scale between them

_____ 11. Provides a means to obtain the opinion of a variety of experts across the country

_____ 12. Observational data recorded using preestablished category systems

_____ 13. Verbal questions asked by the researcher designed before the initiation of data collection

_____ 14. Method in which researcher asks broad question such as "Describe for me your experience with . . ."

PUZZLES

Word Scramble

Directions: Unscramble the sentence below by rearranging the letters to form actual words. Note: You will use all the letters in every word.

Ni slubiphgin eht stulers fo a slogiochipy dusty, eth steaumemen thinquece desen ot eb brisedced ni bonedricales laited.

Secret Message

Directions: Translate the secret message below by substituting one letter for another. For example, if you decide that "b" should really be "d," then "b" will be "d" every time it appears in this puzzle. Hint: Try to translate short words first to establish vowel patterns.

Ksgqilfhzkcfa nfhqwkizqg gxkjvu sq bjhjfaap qntajgzlq

EXERCISES IN CRITIQUE

Directions: Review the Zalon (2004) and the Sethares and Elliott (2004) articles in Appendix B and answer the following questions.

1. For each of the two studies, first identify the measures used; then critique the thoroughness with which each method of measurement was described. In making this judgment, look for the following data about the measurement method: (a) developer of the method of measurement, (b) date measurement method was developed, (c) detailed description of method of measurement (e.g., number of items in scale or steps of performing a physiologic measure), and (d) range of values possible using the measure.

Zalon Study

a. Measure _____

   Critique:

b. Measure _____

   Critique:

c. Measure _____

   Critique:

d. Measure _____

   Critique:

e. Measure _____

   Critique:

Sethares and Elliott Study

a. Measure _____

   Critique:

b. Measure _____

   Critique:

c. Measure _____

   Critique:

CHAPTER 17

Collecting and Managing Data

INTRODUCTION

Read Chapter 17 and then complete the following exercises. These exercises will assist you in learning relevant terms and identifying and critiquing measurement and data collection procedures in published studies. The answers to these exercises are in Appendix A.

RELEVANT TERMS

Directions: Define the following terms in your own words without looking at your text. Then check your definitions with those in the glossary of your text. Using this strategy, you can identify elements of the term that are not yet clear in your mind. Reread the relevant section of the chapter to clarify your understanding of the term.

1. Cleaning data

2. Codebook

3. Coding

4. Computerized database

5. Cost factors

6. Data coding sheet

7. Data collection

8. Data collection forms

9. Data collection plan

10. Data collection problems

11. Data collection tasks

12. Decision points

13. Direct costs

137

14. Indirect costs

15. Input of data

16. Research support systems

17. Serendipity

18. Subject mortality

19. Supportive relationships

20. Time factors

KEY IDEAS

Directions: Provide the appropriate responses.

1. List three decision points during the data collection phase of a study.

   a.

   b.

   c.

2. Describe three situations that might affect consistency in data collection.

   a.

   b.

   c.

3. List four direct costs related to data collection and management.

   a.

   b.

   c.

   d.

4. List three indirect costs related to data collection and management.

a.

b.

c.

5. List five tasks of the researcher during data collection.

a.

b.

c.

d.

e.

MAKING CONNECTIONS

1. Identify three problems with the following planned method of coding data: ages classified into these categories—under 18, 19-45, 45-65, over 65.

a.

b.

c.

2. Identify the problems with the plan for coding data in each of the following questions:

a. From the following list, identify those members of your family who had the flu last year: mother, father, sister, brother, husband, wife, child (coding planned: 1-mother, 2-father, 3-sister, 4-brother, 5-husband, 6-wife, 7-child).

Problems:

b. List the name and dosage of drugs administered for nausea and vomiting.

Problems:

c. List length of hospital admission for each family member (plan is to code by number of days).

Problems:

d. Did you vote last year? _____ Yes _____ No _____ Uncertain

Problems:

PUZZLES

Word Scramble

Directions: Unscramble the sentence below by rearranging the letters to form actual words. Note: You will use all the letters in every word.

Plembors nac eb creipeved rethie sa a trustifanor ro sa a leachleng.

Secret Message

Directions: Translate the secret message below by substituting one letter for another. For example, if you decide that "m" should really be "t," then "m" will be "t" every time it appears in this puzzle. Hint: Try to translate short words first to establish vowel patterns.

Rl bycmpryn fby nw gqwyn, rm grxx, byh bm mpj gwqom uwqqrdxj mrzj.

Crossword Puzzle

Directions: Complete the crossword puzzle below. Note: If the answer is more than one word, there are no blank spaces left between the words.

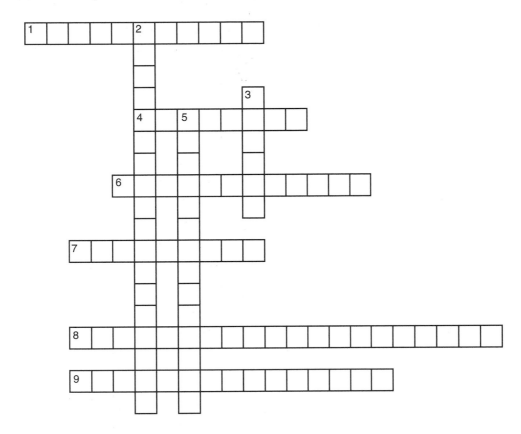

Across

1. The accidental discovery of something valuable or useful during the conduct of a study.
4. Identifies and defines each variable in a study and its range for possible numerical values.
6. Checking raw data to determine errors in data recording, coding, or entry and correct them.
7. Subjects drop out of a study before completion

8. An electronic structured compilation of information that can be scanned, retrieved, or analyzed by computer.
9. A paper form designed to record or scale data for rapid entry into a computer.

Down

2. Details of how data for a study will be implemented and data collected.
3. Process of transforming qualitative data into numerical symbols
5. Precise, systematic gathering of information relevant to research

EXERCISES IN CRITIQUE

Directions: Review the Zalon (2004) and Sethares and Elliott (2004) studies in Appendix B and answer the following questions.

1. In Zalon's study, what is the description of the data collection process? What inconsistencies, if any, do you see in the measurements? Can you identify any threats to the validity of the measures?

2. In Sethares and Elliott's study, what is the description of the data collection process? What inconsistencies, if any, do you see in the measurements? Can you identify any threats to the validity of the measures?

GOING BEYOND

Develop coding sheets for data from the two quantitative studies in Appendix B.

CHAPTER 18

Introduction to Statistical Analysis

INTRODUCTION

Read Chapter 18 and then complete the following exercises. These exercises will assist you in learning relevant terms and identifying and critiquing statistics or results sections of published studies. The answers to these exercises are in Appendix A.

RELEVANT TERMS

Directions: Define the following terms in your own words without looking at your text. Then check your definitions with those in the glossary of your text. Using this strategy, you can identify elements of the term that are not yet clear in your mind. Reread the relevant section of the chapter to clarify your understanding of the term. Note: Understanding the definitions of the terms below is critical to your understanding of the next six chapters of this text.

1. Alpha

2. Asymmetrical

3. Bimodal

4. Calculated variables

5. Causality

6. Central limit theorem

7. Clinical significance

8. Confidence interval

9. Confirmatory analysis

10. Decision theory

11. Degrees of freedom (df)

12. Distribution

13. Estimator

143

14. Exploratory analysis

15. Generalize

16. Infer

17. Inference

18. Interval estimate

19. Kurtosis

20. Leptokurtic

21. Level of significance

22. Mesokurtic

23. Modality

24. Nonparametric statistic

25. Normal curve

26. One-tailed test of significance

27. Parameter

28. Parametric statistic

29. Platykurtic

30. Point estimate

31. Post hoc analysis

32. Power

33. Power analysis

34. Probability theory

35. Relationship

36. Sampling distribution

37. Sampling error

38. Skewed

39. Skewness

40. Standardized score

41. Statistic

42. Symmetry

43. Tailedness

44. Tails

45. Transform

46. Transformed data

47. Two-tailed test of significance

48. Type I error

49. Type II error

50. Unimodal

51. Z score

KEY IDEAS
Directions: Provide the appropriate responses.

1. List eight purposes for the use of statistics.

    a.

    b.

    c.

    d.

e.

f.

g.

h.

2. List the six steps of the process of data analysis.

a.

b.

c.

d.

e.

f.

3. List four activities of data cleaning.

a.

b.

c.

d.

MAKING CONNECTIONS

Directions: Match each term with its definition.

Terms

a. Exploratory analysis
b. Outliers
c. Probability

d. Inference
e. Generalization
f. Type I error

g. Type II error
h. Power
i. Decision theory

Definitions

_____ 1. Accepts null hypothesis when it is false

_____ 2. The probability that a statistical test will detect a significant difference that exists

_____ 3. Conclusion based on evidence

_____ 4. Information applied to population that has been acquired from a specific instance

_____ 5. Rejects null hypothesis when it is true

_____ 6. The likelihood of an event occurring in a given situation

_____ 7. Assumption of no difference

_____ 8. Subjects with extreme values

_____ 9. Descriptive examination of the data

Directions: Match the categories listed below with the statements that follow. Note: You will use some categories more than once.

Categories

a. Decision theory statement
b. Probability theory statement

c. Inference
d. Generalization

Statements

_____ 1. "This finding indicates that subjects with higher levels of self-esteem used more problem-focused coping than did subjects with lower levels of self-esteem" (O'Brien, 1993, p. 57).

_____ 2. "The finding that self-esteem is significantly related to problem-focused coping lends support to the premise of this study that individuals who believe they are persons of value and worth have confidence in themselves and thus are more likely to employ problem-focused strategies" (O'Brien, 1993, p. 58).

_____ 3. "The experimental treatment group will have a more positive perception of the birth experience than the control treatment group at one to two days postpartum" (Fawcett, Pollio, Tully, Baron, Henlkein, & Jones, 1993, p. 50).

_____ 4. "The difference in mean scores between the treatment groups for perception of the birth experience did not reach the required .05 level of significance, $F(1,104) = 3.76$, $p = .055$" (Fawcett, Pollio, Tully, Baron, Henlkein, & Jones, 1993, p. 52).

_____ 5. "The hypotheses were based on the Roy Adaptation Model proposition that management of contextual stimuli promotes adaptation. The study findings provide no support for this proposition, and, therefore, raise a question regarding the credibility of the model" (Fawcett, Pollio, Tully, Baron, Henlkein, & Jones, 1993, p. 52).

_____ 6. "Gastric and intestinal placement of feeding tubes can be differentiated by testing the pH of aspirates from the tubes with a pH-meter (p. 326). . . . Discriminant function analysis provided further support for this hypothesis. . . . There were 85.2% correct classifications overall, with 80.2% of the 405 gastric aspirates correctly classified and 90.5% of the 389 intestinal aspirates correctly classified (p. 327)" (Metheny, Reed, Wiersema, McSweeney, Wehrle, & Clark, 1993, p. 324).

_____ 7. "Using the protocol described in this study, the pH testing method can predict feeding tube position in the gastrointestinal tract with a relatively high degree of accuracy" (Metheny, Reed, Wiersema, McSweeney, Wehrle, & Clark, 1993, p.329).

Directions: For each of the following statistical reports, indicate whether the results were significant or not significant, assuming a level of significance set at 0.05.

Significance

a. Significant
b. Not significant

Statistical Reports

_____ 1. The study evaluated the effectiveness of normal saline versus normal saline containing 10 units per 1 ml heparin for preventing loss of an intermittent intravenous site (heparin lock). Patency of two groups (one with heparin and one without heparin) was examined at 24 hours ($p = 0.75$), 48 hours ($p = 1.00$), and 72 hours ($p = 0.64$) (Shoaf & Oliver, 1992, p. 9).

_____ 2. The study examined interpretations of blood glucose monitoring strips (BGMS) by patients and registered nurses (RNs) experienced in strip use. A one-way Analysis of Variance (ANOVA) was used to examine differences between meter readings, mean patient interpretations, and two of the three RNs ($t[31] = 2.75$, $p = 0.003$; $t[31] = 2.26$, $p = 0.001$; $t[31] = 4.39$, $p < 0.0001$) (Wakefield, Wakefield, & Booth, 1992, p.13).

_____ 3. The study examined the safety and efficacy of 2% nitroglycerin ointment to facilitate venous cannulation. The nitroglycerin ointment is proposed to dilate veins and thus facilitate venous access, but few studies have been conducted to test the proposition. Vein size was measured before and after application of the nitroglycerin ointment or a placebo ointment. Differences between the placebo and nitroglycerin groups were tested using ANOVA ($F_{1,154} = 0.96$, $p = 0.33$) (Griffith, James, & Cropp, 1994, p. 203)

PUZZLES

Word Scramble
Directions: Unscramble the sentence below by rearranging the letters to form actual words. Note: You will use all the letters in every word.

Ot eb fuelus, het decineve morf taad yalinass stum eb lulefarcy maxidene, groznadie, dan venig grnneam.

Secret Message
Directions: Translate the secret message below by substituting one letter for another. For example, if you decide that "s" should really be "v," then "s" will be "v" every time it appears in this puzzle. Hint: Try to translate short words first to establish vowel patterns.

Viwievglivw ger riziv tvszi xlmrkw.

Crossword Puzzle
Directions: Complete the crossword puzzle on the next page. Note: If the answer is more than one word, there are no blank spaces left between the words.

Across

2. A finding sufficiently important to change practice.
4. Cut-off point used to determine whether or not samples are part of the same population.
6. A relatively flat curve with values having large variance among them.
8. Used to determine the risk of a Type II error.
10. A symmetrical, unimodal bell-shaped figure that is a theoretical distribution of all possible scores.
13. Extremes of the normal curve.
15. A curve that is asymmetric.
16. Extend the implications of the findings from the sample to a larger population.
18. Change from one way of expressing to another.
19. An extremely peaked-shaped distribution of a curve.

Down

1. An association of some kind that exists between or among two or more concepts or variables.
3. Use inductive reasoning to move from a specific case to a general statement.
5. Theory that addresses relative rather than absolute causality.
7. The degree of peakedness of a curve reflecting the spread of scores.
9. The independence of a score's value to vary, given other existing score values and their sum.
11. A normal curve.
12. A calculated numerical value of a sample used to estimate a parameter.
14. A measure or numerical value of a population.
17. Descriptive analyses performed to become familiar with the data.

Across

20. Spread of values in a data set.
22. The difference between a sample statistic and a parameter.
23. Statistical tests designed to determine the location of differences in studies with more than two groups.
24. Evenness or balance in a relationship.

Down

21. A distribution with two modes.

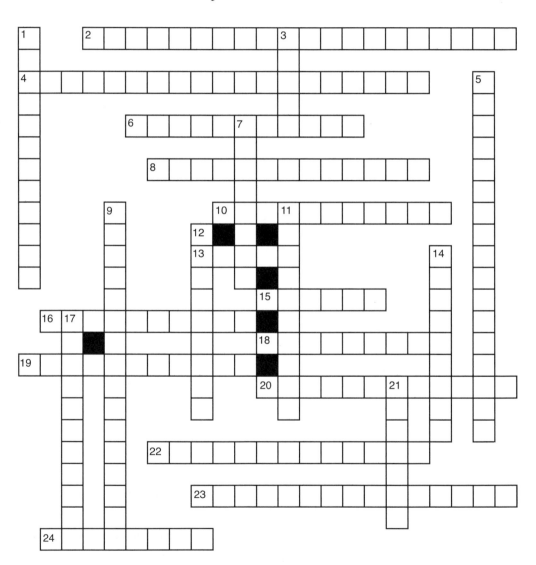

CHAPTER 19

Using Statistics to Describe Variables

INTRODUCTION

Read Chapter 19 and then complete the following exercises. These exercises will assist you in learning relevant terms, identifying and critiquing the descriptive and exploratory statistics in the results sections of published studies, and using these analysis techniques in analyzing data. The answers to these exercises are in Appendix A.

Relevant Terms

Directions: Define the following terms in your own words without looking at your text. Then check your definitions with those in the glossary of your text. Using this strategy, you can identify elements of the term that are not yet clear in your mind. Reread the relevant section of the chapter to clarify your understanding of the term.

1. Autoregressive integrated moving average (ARIMA)

2. Average

3. Bimodal

4. Bland and Altman plots

5. Box-and-whisker plots

6. Central tendency

7. Confidence intervals

8. Descriptive statistics

9. Deterministic component

10. Deviation score

11. Difference scores

12. Dispersion

13. Distribution

151

14. Error in identifying variables

15. Execution errors

16. Exploratory data analysis

17. Far out

18. Fences

19. Forecasting

20. Frequencies

21. Frequency distribution

22. Grouped frequency distribution

23. Hinges

24. Hinge number summary

25. Homogeneity

26. Heterogeneity

27. Inherent variability

28. Kurtosis

29. Least-squares principle

30. Leptokurtic

31. Mean

32. Measure of central tendency

33. Measure of dispersion

34. Measurement error

35. Median

36. Mesokurtic

37. Modal percentage

38. Modality

39. Mode

40. Noise

41. Outliers

42. Outside

43. Pattern

44. Percentage distribution

45. Platykurtic

46. Q plots

47. Random shock

48. Range

49. Residual analysis

50. Scatter plots

51. Standard deviation

52. Stationairty

53. Stem-and-leaf displays

54. Stochastic

55. Sum of squares

56. Summary statistics

57. Survival analysis

58. Symmetry plots

59. Time series analysis

60. Ungrouped frequency distribution

61. Unimodal

62. Variance

63. White noise

KEY IDEAS

Directions: Fill in the blanks or provide the appropriate responses.

1. Descriptive statistics may be the only approach to analysis of data in _____ studies.

2. The first strategy used to organize the data for examination is usually

   _____.

3. Most studies have some categorical data that are presented in the form of

   _____.

4. Any method of grouping results in _____.

5. _____ are particularly useful in comparing the present data with findings from other studies that have varying sample sizes.

6. _____ give some indication of how scores in a sample are dispersed around the mean.

7. A common strategy used to allow meaningful mathematical manipulation of difference in

   scores is to _____.

8. The square root of the variance is called the _____.

9. _____ are a way of comparing a score in one distribution with a score in another distribution.

10. _____ are usually expressed as (38.6,41.4), with 38.6 being the lower end of the interval and 41.4 being the upper end of the interval.

11. _____ is designed to detect the unexpected in the data and to avoid overlooking crucial patterns that may exist.

12. Extreme values, hinges, and fences are terms used to describe elements of

    _____.

13. Individual values that vary from the line of best fit are referred to as _____.

14. A _____ is a common way to illustrate graphically the relationship of two variables.

15. List three statistical strategies used to describe the sample.

    a.

    b.

    c.

MAKING CONNECTIONS
Directions: Perform the following exercises.

Significant Differences
In testing for significant differences between groups, the researcher is determining whether the experimental group belongs to the same population as the control group. An initial step in this process is to compare the mean and standard deviation of the control group with those of the experimental group. The normal curve can be used to visually depict differences in these measures between the two groups. For example, Maloni, Chance, Zhang, Cohen, Betts, and Gange (1993) compared the physical and psychosocial side effects of antepartum hospital complete bed rest, partial bed rest, and no bed rest. Using the no-bed rest group as the control group, we can compare these three groups. For the variable of weight gain, the no-bed rest group mean (M) was 14.48 with a standard deviation (SD) of 4.94. Using this information, the distribution of weight gain in the no-bed rest group can be illustrated.

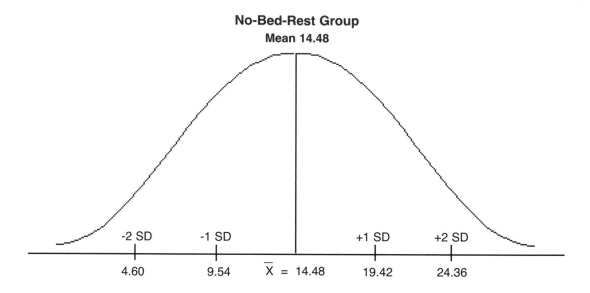

No-Bed-Rest Group
Mean 14.48

-2 SD   -1 SD   +1 SD   +2 SD

4.60   9.54 $\overline{X}$ = 14.48   19.42   24.36

1. The mean for the partial-bed rest group was 10.90, with a standard deviation of 5.29. Using the following curve, illustrate the distribution of values as shown above.

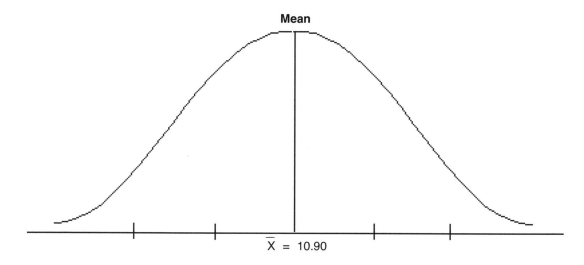

Mean

$\overline{X}$ = 10.90

2. The mean for the complete-bed rest group was 8.17, with a standard deviation of 2.09. Using the following curve, illustrate the distribution of values.

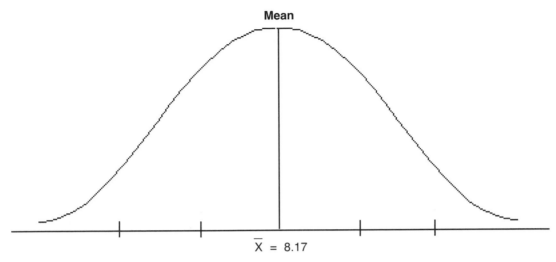

Mean

$\overline{X} = 8.17$

Statistical analyses are required to determine whether the differences in weight gain in the three groups indicate that the groups represent different populations. Analysis of variance (ANOVA) results were F = 7.79, with df = 2.28 and p = .0002, indicating that the groups are significantly different.

PUZZLES

Word Scramble
Directions: Unscramble the sentence below by rearranging the letters to form actual words. Note: You will use all the letters in every word.

Gusni emasreus fo laertnc tencedny ot cebirsed het uatern fo eht aatd soebrsuc eht ticmpa fo emxetre vsluae ro fo veditanois ni het taad.

Secret Message

Directions: Translate the secret message below by substituting one letter for another. For example, if you decide that "t" should really be "g," then "t" will be "g" every time it appears in this puzzle. Hint: Try to translate short words first to establish vowel patterns.

Wzgz zmzobhrh yvtrrnh drgs wvhxirkgrev hgzgrhgrxh rm zmb hgfwb rm dsrxs

gsv wzgz ziv mfnvirx, rmxofwrmt hlnv jfzorgzgrev hgfwrvh.

Crossword Puzzle

Directions: Complete the crossword puzzle on the next page. Note: If the answer is more than one word, there are no blank spaces left between the words.

Across

1. Values beyond the inner fence in stem-and-leaf analyses.
3. The difference between what exists in reality and what is measured.
8. Value obtained by summing all the scores and dividing that total by the number of scores being summed.
11. Extreme values in a set of data that are exceptions to the overall findings.
14. Value that occurs with greatest frequency.
17. Designed to analyze repeated measures from a given time until a certain event occurs.
21. Used to identify outliers.
22. List of all measures of a variable.
23. Random variance in the data in time-series analysis.
24. A repetitive, regular, or continuous occurrence in time-series analysis.
25. Distribution of values.
26. An analysis of deviation values in a data set.

Down

2. The square root of the variance.
4. Using differencing to make data homogeneous.
5. Exploratory data analysis technique.
6. Designed to detect the unexpected in the data.
7. Naturally expected random observations in the extreme ends of the tail.
9. Values displayed by quartile.
10. The score at the exact center of an ungrouped frequency distribution.
12. Projects results of ARIMA modeling into the future.
13. Distribution of categorical data.
15. Obtained by subtracting the mean from the raw score.
16. Values beyond the outer fence.
18. A graphic illustration of the point at which each value of x and y intersect.
19. Result obtained by adding the squares of difference scores.
20. A value halfway from each extreme to the median in a stem-and-leaf display.

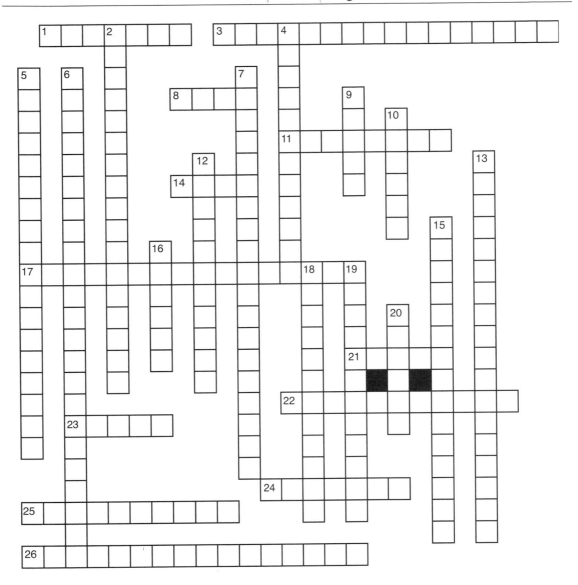

EXERCISES IN CRITIQUE

Directions: Review the two quantitative studies in Appendix B—Zalon (2004) and Sethares and Elliott (2004)—and answer the following questions.

1. Identify the descriptive analyses performed in the Zalon study. What analyses were not reported that you believe should have been included? Why would this information be important to report? Identify exploratory data analyses performed in the study.

2. Identify the descriptive analyses performed in the Sethares and Elliott study. What analyses were not reported that you believe should have been included? Why would this information be important to report? Identify exploratory data analyses performed in the study.

GOING BEYOND

Using the data set below, create a stem-and-leaf display and a box-and-whisker plot.

23, 15, 36, 37, 5, 62, 356, 32, 37, 3, 44, 52, 456, 2, 5, 2, 54, 24, 25, 26, 38, 58, 43, 36, 97, 46, 35, 35, 34, 4, 5, 75, 4, 89, 6, 8, 3, 7, 35, 5, 3, 6, 58, 76, 5, 8, 45, 3, 6, 33, 65, 87, 58, 45, 35, 35, 24, 23, 11, 35, 24, 26, 3, 35, 26, 3, 78, 5, 8, 5, 9, 3, 66, 36, 36, 26, 35, 37, 42, 63, 43, 21, 45

Using Statistics to Examine Relationships

INTRODUCTION

Read Chapter 20 and then complete the following exercises. These exercises will assist you in understanding and critiquing bivariate inferential statistics in the results sections of published studies and in conducting these analysis techniques using study data. The answers to these exercises are in Appendix A.

RELEVANT TERMS

Directions: Define the following terms in your own words without looking at your text. Then check your definitions with those in the glossary of your text. Using this strategy, you can identify elements of the term that are not yet clear in your mind. Reread the relevant section of the chapter to clarify your understanding of the term.

1. Additive relationships

2. Beta weights

3. Bivariate correlation

4. Canonical correlation

5. Causal flow

6. Causal pathway

7. Causal relationships

8. Coefficient

9. Communality

10. Confirmatory factor analysis

11. Correlational analysis

12. Correlational matrix

13. Cross-lagged panel correlation

14. Curvilinear relationship

15. Cutoff point

16. Eigenvalues

17. Endogeneous variables

18. Estimation

19. Exogenous variables

20. Exploratory factor analysis

21. Factor

22. Factor analysis

23. Factor loading

24. Factor rotation

25. Factor score

26. Fixed parameters

27. Free variables

28. Goodness of fit

29. Homoscedastic

30. Inverse linear relationship

31. Kendall's tau

32. Latent variables

33. Linear composite

34. Linear relationship

35. Loadings

36. Magnitude of relationship

37. Multivariate correlations

38. Negative linear relationship

39. Noncausal correlations

40. Nonlinear relationship

41. Oblique rotation

42. Path coefficient

43. Pearson's product-moment correlation

44. Percentage of variance

45. Perfect correlation

46. Positive linear relationship

47. Principal components factor analysis

48. Regression line

49. Residual variables

50. Respecification

51. Scatter diagram

52. Scree test

53. Secondary loading

54. Spearman rho

55. Specification

56. Spurious correlation

57. Strength of relationship

58. Structural equation modeling

59. Symmetrical relationship

60. Validation

61. Varimax rotation

62. Weak correlation

63. Weighting

KEY IDEAS

Directions: Fill in the blanks in the following sentences.

1. The purpose of correlational analyses is to identify _____ between or among variables.

2. In correlational analyses, all of the data are obtained from _____ group(s).

3. When correlational analyses are planned, sampling and data collection should be designed to

   maximize the possibility of obtaining the _____ of possible values on each variable in the study.

4. A _____ is the line that best represents the values of the raw scores plotted on a scatter diagram.

5. In a negative linear relationship, a _____ score on one variable is related to a

   _____ score on the other variable.

6. _____ data will provide the best information when using correlational analyses.

7. _____ is used when performing correlational analyses on nominal data.

8. Correlational analysis provides information about whether the relationships are

   _____ or _____ and also the _____ of the relationship.

9. The data are _____ before conducting the analysis when performing correlational analysis using ordinal data.

10. Performing bivariate correlational analyses on every pair of variables in a data set will provide

    a _____.

11. _____ correlations are relationships between variables that are not logical.

12. _____ examines interrelationships among large numbers of variables.

13. The purpose of canonical correlation is to analyze the relationships between _____ or more dependent variables and _____ or more independent variables.

14. Structural equation modeling tests _____.

MAKING CONNECTIONS

Directions: Match each term with its definition.

Terms

a. Scree
b. Symmetrical relationship
c. Factor loading
d. Negative relationship
e. Residual variable
f. Curvilinear relationship

g. Percentage of variance explained
h. Bivariate correlation
i. Factor analysis
j. Develop scales
k. Eigenvalue
l. Positive relationship

m. Communality
n. Test theory
o. Factor
p. Small sample
q. Path coefficient
r. Degree of relationship

Definitions

_____   1.   Cluster of variables linked together
_____   2.   Extent single variable related to cluster of variables
_____   3.   Scores vary together (in same direction)
_____   4.   Test used to determine number of factors
_____   5.   The extent of linear relationship between 2 variables
_____   6.   Cannot be examined with correlational analysis
_____   7. r^2
_____   8.   High correlation can be nonsignificant
_____   9.   Aids in identifying theoretical constructs
_____ 10.   Factor analysis
_____ 11.   Sum of squared weights for a factor
_____ 12.   Direction of linear relationship cannot be determined
_____ 13.   Amount of variance in variable explained by all factors
_____ 14.   Structural equation modeling
_____ 15. r
_____ 16.   Scores vary in opposite directions from each other
_____ 17.   Indicates the effect of an independent variable on a dependent variable
_____ 18.   Not explained within the theory

McNee and McCabe (2004)

Directions: In the following statistical report, indicate the strength of the correlation and whether the results were significant, assuming a level of significance set at 0.05. Use a highlighter to mark significant relationships. A space has been left after each value for you to indicate the strength of the relationship. Indicate H for high, M for moderate, and L for low.

McNee and McCabe (2004). The transtheoretical model of behavior change and smokers in southern Appalachia, *Nursing Research*, 54(4), 243-250. [The study was supported by a grant from the National Institute of Nursing Research.]

Objective: To identify, by examining the applicability of the transtheoretical model for southern Appalachian smokers, the percentage of individuals in each of the five stages of change, the use of the processes of change from the transtheoretical model, and the scores on recognized predictors of smoking cessation including the temptation to smoke, the perceived barriers to cessation, the pros and cons of smoking, and nicotine dependence. (p. 243)

Nicotine dependence was significantly correlated with the pros of smoking scores ($r = 0.37$;

$p < .001$), _____ barriers to smoking ($r = .32$; $p < 0.001$), _____ and temptation scores ($r = .46$;

$p. < 0.001$), _____ supporting the theoretical relations proposed in the TTM. However, the levels of nicotine dependence did not vary significantly across the stages of change.

Gary and Yarandi (2004)

Directions: Review the statistical report below and answer the questions that follow.

Gary and Yarandi (2004). Depression among southern rural African American women. *Nursing Research*, 54(4), 251-259.

An iterated principal-factor analysis was performed, in which squared multiple correlations were used for the initial communality estimates, and a Promax (oblique) rotation was used to identify the self-reported dimensions of depression. The minimum 80% variance criterion and the scree plot were used to determine the optimal number of factors. . . . . Two factors were extracted. . . . The coefficient alphas for the factors suggested that the first two common factors were potentially reliable for this sample. The coefficient alphas for the two factors were 0.98 and 0.83, respectively. The two extracted factors explained 89% of the common variance. Two comparably sized eigenvalues of 5.35 and 5.53 were found for the reduced correlation matrix, and the correlation between the two oblique factors was 0.57 ($p < 0.001$). . . . Symptoms such as pessimism, worthlessness, punishment feelings, sadness, self-dislike, loss of interest, indecisiveness, and past failure tended to load high on the first factor. All these symptoms were psychological and cognitive in nature. Therefore, Factor I was a cognitive dimension of self-reported depression. Factor II explained somatic symptoms such as tiredness or fatigue, loss of energy, concentration difficulty, irritability, changes in appetite, changes in sleeping pattern, loss of interest in sex, and loss of pleasure. Such factors were thought to represent a "somatic-affective" dimension of self-reported depression.

1. Highlight the terms related to factor analysis that you recognize. Examine the results. Interpret the results based on your understanding of factor analysis.

PUZZLES

Word Scramble

Directions: Unscramble the sentence below by rearranging the letters to form actual words. Note: You will use all the letters in every word.

Kawe larrastoonic yam eb rompitnat hewn mobdince thiw roeth blaivarse

Secret Message

Directions: Translate the secret message below by substituting one letter for another. For example, if you decide that "e" should really be "p," then "e" will be "p" every time it appears in this puzzle. Hint: Try to translate short words first to establish vowel patterns.

Ra eijebibmrca lci fciijxbmrcabx babxkrk, hbmb fcxxjfrca kmibmjnrjk kpcoxh dj

exbaajh mc zburzryj mpj eckkrdrxrmw cl cdmbraran mpj loxx ibanj cl eckkrdxj

qbxojk ca jbfp qbirbdxj mc dj okjh ra mpj babxwkrk.

Crossword Puzzle

Directions: Complete the crossword puzzle. Note: If the answer is more than one word, there are no blank spaces left between the words.

Across

1. A two-dimensional plot designed to illustrate the relationship between two variables.
5. A procedure designed to obtain the best fit of variables to factors.
6. _____ (relationship)—increases as the correlation value moves away from zero.
7. Indicates the extent a variable is related to the cluster of variables.
10. _____ correlation—a relationship between two variables that makes no sense.
14. _____ variables—caused by elements outside the theory being tested.
15. A cluster of variables linked closely together.
17. _____ variable—not measurable by direct observation; may be composed of several variables combined
18. _____ correlation—a relationship below 0.3.
19. The extent to which the variable is correlated with the factor.
20. Equal variance on each side of the line of best fit.
21. _____ correlation—test of relationship between two variables.
22. _____ variables—elements external to a theory that are related to variables within the theory.
23. Multiplying the variable score by the factor loading.

Down

2. In path analysis, how well the resulting model fits the data.
3. A nonlinear relationship.
4. Sum of the squared weights for each factor.
6. Used to determine the number of factors to set in a factor analysis.
8. _____ relationship—a relationship value greater than zero.
9. The effect of the independent variable on the dependent variable in structural equation modeling.
11. A type of factor rotation in which factors are allowed to be correlated.
12. The line that best represents the values plotted on a scattergram.
13. _____ variables—those variables whose variations are explained within the theory being studied.
16. _____ correlation—test of relationship among multiple independent and dependent variables.

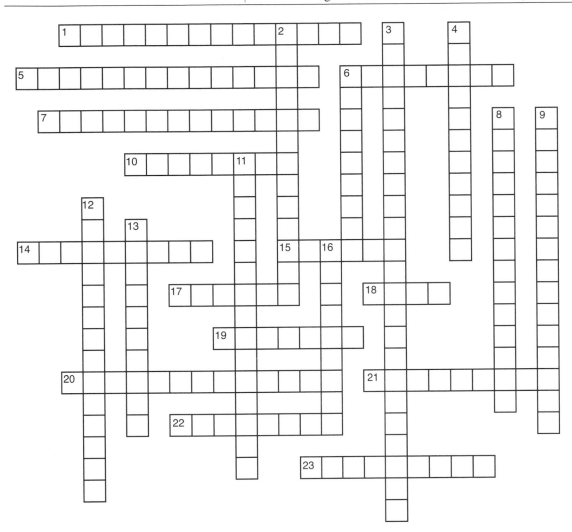

GOING BEYOND

Identify a recently published study using correlation, factor analysis, or structural equation modeling. Read the study and highlight terms in the study that you are familiar with from this chapter. In the results section, identify and circle significant results. Identify the results with the greatest strength. Match your findings with those of the author in the findings section.

CHAPTER 21

Using Statistics to Predict

INTRODUCTION

Read Chapter 21 and then complete the following exercises. These exercises will assist you in understanding and critiquing bivariate inferential statistics in the results sections of published studies and in conducting these analysis techniques using study data. The answers to these exercises are in Appendix A.

RELEVANT TERMS

Directions: Define the following terms in your own words without looking at your text. Then check your definitions with those in the glossary of your text. Using this strategy, you can identify elements of the term that are not yet clear in your mind. Reread the relevant section of the chapter to clarify your understanding of the term.

1. Backward stepwise regression

2. Bivariate

3. Beta score

4. Coefficient of determination

5. Confirmatory regression analysis

6. Cross-validation

7. Curvilinear

8. Discriminant analysis

9. Discriminant function

10. Dummy variables

11. Estimate

12. Exploratory regression analysis

13. Forward stepwise regression

14. Hierarchical regression

15. Holdout sample

16. Homoscedasticity

17. Horizontal axis

18. Intercept

19. Line of best fit

20. Linear discriminant function (LDF)

21. Linear relationship

22. Logistic regression

23. Logit analysis

24. Maximum likelihood estimation

25. Method of least squares

26. Multicollinearity

27. Multilevel analysis

28. Multiple regression

29. Multiplicative terms

30. Nonlinearity analysis

31. Partialing out

32. Predicted score

33. Prediction equation

34. Predictive validity

35. Predictor variable

36. Probability

37. Regression

38. Regression coefficient R

39. Regression equation

40. Regression line

41. Residual analysis

42. Residual error

43. Scatter plot

44. Shrinkage of R^2

45. Simple linear regression

46. Simultaneous regression

47. Slope

48. Stepwise regression

49. Structured coefficients

50. Transformed terms

51. Variation

52. Vertical axis

53. Y-intercept

KEY IDEAS

Directions: Fill in the blanks or provide the appropriate responses.

1. The purpose of a regression analysis is to predict or explain as much of the _____ in the value of a dependent variable as possible.

2. Predictive analyses are based on _____ theory.

3. Prediction is one approach to examining _____ relationships.

4. The _____ variable(s) cause(s) variation in the value of the _____ variable.

5. In plotting a regression line, the horizontal axis represents _____ and the vertical axis represents _____.

6. What is the procedure for developing the line of best fit?

7. The outcome of a regression analysis is the regression coefficient _____.

8. R^2 indicates the amount of _____ in the data that is explained by the regression equation.

9. Simple linear regression provides a means to _____ the value of a dependent variable based on the value of an independent variable.

10. Multiple regression analyses are closely related mathematically to

_____ .

11. In multiple regression, more than one _____ variable is entered into the analysis.

12. Multicollinearity can be minimized by careful selection of _____ variables.

13. Multicollinearity causes problems with _____.

14. With multicollinearity, the amount of variance explained by each variable in the equation will

be _____.

15. A _____ of types of variables may be used in a single regression equation.

16. The outcome of a regression analysis is referred to as a _____.

17. Discriminant analysis is designed to predict _____.

18. What are the outcomes of a discriminant function analysis called?

MAKING CONNECTIONS

Regression Analysis

1. List the three assumptions of regression analysis.

   a.

   b.

   c.

2. What is the algebraic equation for a straight line?

3. List four types of variables that can be used in a regression equation.

   a.

   b.

   c.

   d.

4. List five types of regression analyses that can be performed.

   a.

   b.

   c.

   d.

   e.

Directions: Match each term with its description.

Terms

a. Regression equation
b. Line of best fit
c. y intercept
d. b
e. Least squares method

f. Coefficient R
g. t
h. t will increase as
i. t will decrease as
j. Cross-validation

k. ANOVA
l. R^2
m. Multiple regression
n. Shrinkage of R^2
o. Multicollinearity

Descriptions

_____ 1. Amount of variance explained in regression equation
_____ 2. Test of regression equation using new sample
_____ 3. Point where regression line crosses the y-axis
_____ 4. b moves farther from zero
_____ 5. Based on decision theory
_____ 6. Reduces prediction ability of original regression equation
_____ 7. Statistic to test significance of regression equation
_____ 8. Causal proposition
_____ 9. Best explanation of linear relationship between 2 variables
_____ 10. Outcome of regression analysis
_____ 11. Sum of squared deviations increases
_____ 12. The slope
_____ 13. Based on probability theory
_____ 14. Procedure to develop line of best fit
_____ 15. Reduces capacity to generalize regression findings

PUZZLES

Word Scramble
Directions: Unscramble the sentence below by rearranging the letters to form actual words. Note: You will use all the letters in every word.

Eht gloa fo onerigress sainisly si ot mintedeer who trulycarae noe nac dripcet het evual fo a tendneped raibleva dabes no eth aluve ro sualve fo neo ro rome pendnindeet raveblias.

Secret Message

Directions: Translate the secret message below by substituting one letter for another. For example, if you decide that "b" should really be "d," then "b" will be "d" every time it appears in this puzzle. Hint: Try to translate short words first to establish vowel patterns.

Hrofqrzrybym bybxcoro ro hjornyjh mw hjmjqzryj pwg bffkqbmjxc wyj fby

uqjhrfm mpj ibxkj wq ibxkjo wl wyj wq zwqj ryhjujyhjym ibqrbdxjo.

Crossword Puzzle

Directions: Complete the crossword puzzle on the next page. Note: If the answer is more than one word, there are no blank spaces left between the words.

Across

2. All independent variables entered at the same time into a regression analysis.
3. Independent variable.
5. The accuracy of a predictive equation.
10. Predicts group membership.
15. Categorical variables.
17. The X axis.
18. Test of ability of regression equation to predict in a new sample.

Down

1. Analyzes more than one independent variable.
2. b, the coefficient of x.
4. Regression in which the dependent variable is categorical.
6. The Y axis.
7. A straight line drawn through plotted scores that provides the best explanation of the linear relationship between two variables.
8. The product of two terms that expresses the joint effect of both.
9. Best subset of discriminating variables.
11. Sample data not included in first analysis.
12. Equal scatter of values of y above and below the regression.
13. The outcome of a regression analysis.
14. Two variables.
16. The point on the Y axis where the line of best fit interfaces.

EXERCISES IN CRITIQUE

Directions: Review Zalon's study in Appendix B and answer the following questions. Consider the research question for Zalon's study: What is the relation of pain, depression, and fatigue to recovery, as measured by functional status and self-perception of recovery in older adults who have had major abdominal surgery?

1. Below, list the variables that will be used in statistical analyses to answer the research question and the level of measurement of each variable.

Variable   Level of Measurement

2. Zalon performed analysis to examine the possibility of multicollinearity. What was the outcome of this analysis?

3. What form of regression analysis was used in the study?

4. How many regression analyses were performed? Why?

5. State the results of the analysis, providing numerical values.

6. Circle the appropriate categorization of the results.

   a.   Significant and predicted

   b.   Nonsignificant

   c.   Significant and not predicted

   d.   Mixed results

   e.   Unexpected

GOING BEYOND

Search current issues of nursing research journals for studies using regression analyses. Evaluate the adequacy of descriptions of the procedures performed.

CHAPTER 22

Using Statistics to Examine Causality

INTRODUCTION

Read Chapter 22 and then complete the following exercises. These exercises will assist you in understanding and critiquing bivariate inferential statistics in the results sections of published studies and in conducting these analysis techniques using study data. The answers to these exercises are in Appendix A.

RELEVANT TERMS

Directions: Define the following terms in your own words without looking at your text. Then check your definitions with those in the glossary of your text. Using this strategy, you can identify elements of the term that are not yet clear in your mind. Reread the relevant section of the chapter to clarify your understanding of the term.

1. ANCOVA

2. ANOVA

3. ANOVA summary table

4. Asymmetrical analysis

5. Binomial distribution

6. Bonferroni procedure

7. Between groups variance

8. Causality

9. Cell

10. Chi-squared

11. Chi-squared test of independence

12. Cochran Q test

13. Confounding variable

14. Conservative post hoc test

15. Contingency coefficient (C)

16. Contingency table

17. Covariate

18. Cramer's V

19. Critical value

20. Cross-tabulation

21. Cumulative frequency

22. Degrees of freedom

23. Dependent variable

24. Dichotomous

25. Difference score

26. Distribution-free

27. Escalation of significance

28. F statistic

29. Factorial ANOVA

30. False null hypothesis

31. Friedman two-way analysis of variance by ranks

32. Grand mean

33. Grouped frequency

34. Homogeneity of variance

35. Independent samples

36. Independent variable

37. Interaction effects

38. Interval data

39. Intervention effects

40. Kolmogorov-Smirnov two-sample test

41. Kruskal-Wallis one-way analysis of variance

42. Lambda

43. Liberal post hoc test

44. Location of significant difference

45. Magnitude of change

46. Mann-Whitney U test

47. MANOVA

48. McNemar test

49. Multiple covariates

50. Nominal data

51. Nonparametric procedure

52. Observed cell frequency

53. Ordinal data

54. Parametric procedure

55. Partitioning

56. Phi coefficient

57. Pooled variance

58. Post hoc analysis

59. Ranking

60. Related samples

61. Robust to violation of assumptions

62. Robustness

63. Sampling distribution

64. Sign test

65. Standard error

66. Statistical assumptions

67. Statistical control

68. Statistical power

69. Statistical value

70. Sum of squares

71. Sum of squares within

72. Symmetrical analysis

73. t distribution

74. t-test

75. Total sum of squares

76. Total variance

77. Wald-Wolfowitz runs test

78. Wilcoxon matched-pairs signed-ranks test

79. Within groups variance

80. Z distribution

81. Z statistic

KEY IDEAS

Directions: Fill in the blank in the following sentences.

1. If subjects are randomly assigned to treatment and control groups, the groups are

   _____.

2. If subjects serve as their own control by using the pretest as a control, the observations (and

   therefore the groups) are _____.

3. Use of _____ allows visual comparison of summary data output related to two variables within the sample.

4. One assumption of the chi-square test of independence is that there is

   _____ of data for each subject in the sample.

5. The t-test is _____ to moderate violation of its assumptions.

6. ANOVA compares the variance _____ each group with the variance _____ groups.

7. ANOVA is relatively sensitive to variations in _____ between groups.

8. ANCOVA partials out the variance resulting from a confounding variable by performing

   _____ prior to performing ANOV A.

PUZZLES

Word Scramble

Directions: Unscramble the sentence below by rearranging the letters to form actual words. Note: You will use all the letters in every word.

Het t-sett nac eb sued yonl noe emit rundig lanisysa ot mixenea tada mofr wot mapless ni a yustd.

Secret Message

Directions: Translate the secret message below by substituting one letter for another. For example, if you decide that "c" should really be "y," then "c" will be "y" every time it appears in this puzzle. Hint: Try to translate short words first to establish vowel patterns.

Ry zbyc fbojo dribqrbmj bybxcoro hwjo ywm uqwirhj b fxjbq urfmkqj wl mpj

hcybzrfo wl mpj ormkbmrwy

Crossword Puzzle

Directions: Complete the crossword puzzle on the next page. Note: If the answer is more than one word, there are no blank spaces left between the words.

Across

1. A numerical value obtained from a sample.
5. Uses cut-off point to judge significance of differences.
8. Results unlikely due to chance.
11. Probability that an analysis will detect a difference that exists.
12. Exclude incomplete data from analysis.
14. Analysis used to predict the value of one variable if values of other variables are known.
15. Test that uses variance to compare differences between groups.
16. Groups in which selection of one subject is related to selection of another subject.
17. Determines an outcome.
18. Measure of central tendency for interval data.
19. Extreme of the normal curve.
20. Dispersion of values in sample.
21. Difference between lowest value and highest value.
22. Subjects with extreme values unlike the rest of the sample.
23. Measure of central tendency for ordinal data.
24. Outcome of data analysis.
25. Judgment based on evidence.

Down

2. Analysis technique used to determine differences between two samples.
3. Statistical procedures used to examine the data descriptively.
4. Measure of central tendency for nominal data.
5. The spread of the scores around the mean is referred to as the _____ of scores.
6. Sample that is like the population.
7. Meanings of conclusions for the body of nursing knowledge.
9. Theoretical symmetrical distribution of all possible values.
10. Statistical test used to analyze nominal data.
13. Tests performed after initial analyses to identify specific groups that are different.

EXERCISES IN CRITIQUE

Directions: Review Sethares and Elliott's (2004) study in Appendix B and answer the following questions. Consider the hypotheses for Sethares and Elliott's study: (1) Persons who receive the intervention will have lower HF readmission rates. (2) Persons who receive the intervention will report better quality of life. (3) Intervention subjects will report fewer barriers and more benefits to performing self-care of HF after receiving the tailored message intervention.

1. List the variables that will be used in statistical analyses to test hypothesis 1 and identify the level of measurement of each variable.

Variable   Level of Measurement

2. Identify the groups included in the first analysis.

   a.

   b.

3. Are these groups dependent or independent?

4. What statistical procedure was used to test this hypothesis?

5. Why was this procedure chosen?

6. Using the algorithm on page 457 of your text, judge the appropriateness of the statistical procedure used to test hypothesis 1. Can you identify other statistical procedures that might have been better? Write a brief paragraph expressing your judgment.

7. State the results of the first analysis, providing numerical values.

8. From the list below, circle the appropriate categorization of the results you stated in question 7.
   a.   Significant and predicted
   b.   Nonsignificant
   c.   Significant and not predicted
   d.   Mixed results
   e.   Unexpected

9. List the variables that will be used in statistical analyses to test hypothesis 2 and identify the level of measurement of each variable.

Variable   Level of Measurement

10. Identify the groups included in the second analysis.

   a.

   b.

11. Are these groups dependent or independent?

12. What statistical procedure was used to test this hypothesis?

13. Why was this procedure chosen?

14. Using the algorithms on pages 457-458 of your text, judge the appropriateness of the statistical procedure used to test hypothesis 2. Can you identify other statistical procedures that might have been better? Write a brief paragraph expressing your judgment.

15. State the results of the second analysis, providing numerical values.

16. From the list below, circle the appropriate categorization of the results you stated in question 15.
    a. Significant and predicted
    b. Nonsignificant
    c. Significant and not predicted
    d. Mixed results
    e. Unexpected

17. List the variables that will be used in statistical analyses to test hypothesis 3 and the level of measurement of each variable.

Variable   Level of Measurement

18. Identify the groups included in the third analysis.

    a.

    b.

    c.

19. Are these groups dependent or independent?

20. What statistical procedure was used to test this hypothesis?

21. Why was this procedure chosen?

22. Using the algorithm on page 457 of your text, judge the appropriateness of the statistical procedure used to test hypothesis 3. Can you identify other statistical procedures that might have been better? Write a brief paragraph expressing your judgment.

23. State the results of the third analysis, providing numerical values.

24. From the list below, circle the appropriate categorization of the results you stated in question 23.
    a. Significant and predicted
    b. Nonsignificant
    c. Significant and not predicted
    d. Mixed results
    e. Unexpected

GOING BEYOND

Search current issues of nursing research journals for studies using advanced statistical procedures. Evaluate the adequacy of descriptions of the procedures performed.

CHAPTER 23

Qualitative Research Methodology

INTRODUCTION

Read Chapter 23 and then complete the following exercises. These exercises will assist you in learning relevant terms and reading and comprehending published qualitative studies. The answers for these exercises are in Appendix A.

RELEVANT TERMS

Directions: Define the following terms in your own words without looking at your text. Then check your definitions with those in the glossary of your text. Using this strategy, you can identify elements of the term that are not yet clear in your mind. Reread the relevant section of the chapter to clarify your understanding of the term.

1. Analytic induction

2. Auditability

3. Being with

4. Bracketing

5. Case study

6. Causal network

7. Codes

8. Chronolog

9. Coding

10. Cognitive mapping

11. Complete observer

12. Complete participation

13. Conceptual/theoretical Coherence

14. Complete participation

15. Connecting findings to theory

16. Content analysis

17. Context chart

18. Critical incident chart

19. Critical social theory

20. Data-reducing devices

21. Data triangulation

22. Decentering devices

23. Decision trail

24. Descriptive codes

25. Displaying data

26. Dwelling with the data

27. Eliminative induction

28. Enumerative induction

29. Ethical analyses

30. Ethnographic methodology

31. Event-time matrix

32. Explanatory codes

33. Explanatory effects matrix

34. External criticism

35. Factoring

36. Feminist research methods

37. Field research

38. Focus group

39. Foundational inquiries

40. Going native

41. Grounded theory methodology

42. Historical research

43. Immersion in the culture

44. Immersion in the data

45. Internal criticism

46. Interpretation

47. Interpretative codes

48. Intuiting

49. Life story

50. Logical chain of evidence

51. Marginal remarks

52. Matrices

53. Memoing

54. Metaphors

55. Method mixing

56. Moderator

57. Narrative analysis

58. Observer-as-participant

59. Participant-as-observer

60. Participatory research

61. Pattern-making devices

62. Patterns

63. Phenomenological research

64. Philosophical analyses

65. Philosophical studies

66. Premature parsimony

67. Process-outcome matrix

68. Propositions

69. Reflective remarks

70. Reflexive thought

71. Reflexivity

72. Researcher-participant relationships

73. Segmentation

74. Splitting variables

75. Story

76. Storytaker

77. Storytelling

78. Themes

79. Unstructured interview

80. Unstructured observation

81. Variable-specific context chart

KEY IDEAS
Directions: Fill in the blanks or provide the appropriate responses.

1. Qualitative data analysis occurs _____ data collection.

2. Qualitative data analysis uses _____ rather than _____ as the basis for analysis.

3. In qualitative analysis, the flow of reasoning moves from _____ to increasing

   _____.

4. Auditability requires that the researcher establish _____ for categorizing data, arriving at ratings, or making judgments.

5. The researcher's _____ is a key factor in qualitative research.

6. Memos move the researcher toward _____.

7. Findings are often described from the orientation of the _____.

8. List four types of researcher-participant relationships and define them.

   a.

   b.

   c.

   d.

9. List three characteristics of researcher-participant relationships in qualitative research.

   a.

   b.

   c.

10. List four methods of reducing data in qualitative research.

    a.

    b.

c.

d.

11. List six methods of drawing conclusions in analyzing qualitative data.

a.

b.

c.

d.

e.

f.

MAKING CONNECTIONS

Directions: Match the qualitative methodology types listed below with the examples that follow.

Qualitative Methodology Types

a. Phenomenology
b. Grounded theory
c. Ethnography
d. Historical
e. Philosophical
f. Critical social theory

Examples

_____   1. Ask questions that reveal flaws in logic
_____   2. Reveal power relations
_____   3. Check the fit between the emerging theory and the original data
_____   4. Dwell with the data
_____   5. Clarify validity and reliability of data
_____   6. Emergence of the core variable
_____   7. Acquire informants
_____   8. Develop an inventory of sources
_____   9. Intuiting
_____   10. Search for negative instances of categories
_____   11. Gaining entrance
_____   12. Examination of principles to guide conduct
_____   13. Analysis of constraints on human action

_____ 14. Use archival data
_____ 15. I-Thou being with the participant
_____ 16. Avoid "going native"
_____ 17. Questions more important than answers

PUZZLES

Word Scramble
Directions: Unscramble the sentence below by rearranging the letters to form actual words. Note: You will use all the letters in every word.

Salyasin squirere scros-hicknecg heac tib fo taad thiw lal het throe stib fo adat.

Secret Message
Directions: Translate the secret message below by substituting one letter for another. For example, if you decide that "t" should really be "q," then "t" will be "q" every time it appears in this puzzle. Hint: Try to translate short words first to establish vowel patterns.

Rqh ipsruwdqw gliihuhqfh ehhwzhhk txdqwlwdwlyh dqg txdolwdwlyh uhvhdufk

lv wkh qdwxuh ri uhodwlrqvklsv ehwzhhq wkh uhvhdufkhu dqg wkh iqglylgxdov

ehlqj vwxglhg.

Crossword Puzzle

Directions: Complete the crossword puzzle on the next page. Note: If the answer is more than one word, there are no blank spaces left between the words.

Across

2. Explanation.
5. Developing graphic map of concepts and relationships.
9. Divide into parts.
11. Intensive exploration of a single unit of study.
12. Tale.
14. Have a feeling.
15. Decreasing volume of information.
16. Suspending or laying aside what is known.
17. Person who hears a study.
18. Making written note of.
19. Instructive.
20. Rigorous development of a decision trail.
21. Developing categories.

Down

1. Interaction between self and data.
3. Reducing categories too soon.
4. Relating a study.
6. Premises.
7. Method of retracing choices.
8. _____ (with)—abiding.
10. Involve oneself.
13. Using a combination of methods.

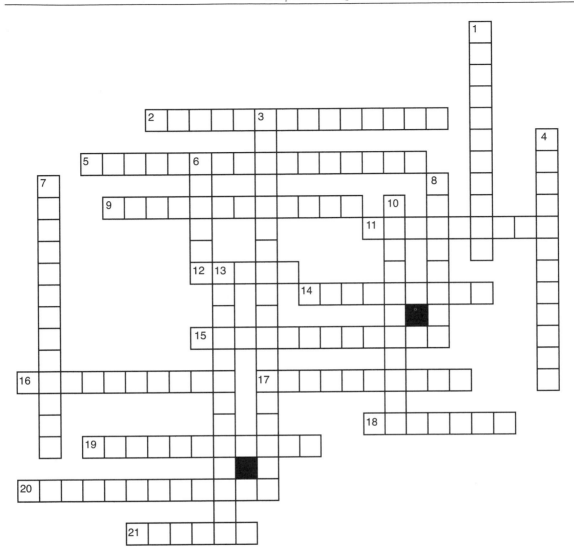

EXERCISES IN CRITIQUE

Directions: Read the Wright (2003) article in Appendix A and answer the following questions.

1. Identify the philosophical base of the study.

2. Describe the methodology using to collect and analyze the data.

3. Did the philosophical base influence the selection of methods?

4. How well did the researcher follow the methodology?

5. Can you follow the author's logic in developing conclusions from the study?

6. What flaws do you see in the study?

7. How could the information from this study be used clinically?

GOING BEYOND

Identify full-text qualitative studies in CINAHL. Read them and identify the methodology used in each study. How well do you think the researcher(s) did in following the methodology? What flaws do you see in each study?

CHAPTER 24

Interpreting Research Outcomes

INTRODUCTION

Read Chapter 24 and then complete the following exercises. These exercises will assist you in learning relevant terms and identifying and critiquing the discussion sections of published studies. The answers to these exercises are in Appendix A.

RELEVANT TERMS

Directions: Define the following terms in your own words without looking at your text. Then check your definitions with those in the glossary of your text. Using this strategy, you can identify elements of the term that are not yet clear in your mind. Reread the relevant section of the chapter to clarify your understanding of the term.

1. Conclusions

2. Empirical generalization

3. Examining evidence

4. Findings

5. Generalization

6. Implications

7. Interpretation

8. Landmark studies

9. Mixed results

10. Negative results

11. Nonsignificant results

12. Practical significance

13. Results

201

14. Significance of findings

15. Significant and not predicted results

16. Significant and predicted results

17. Statistical significance

18. Suggestions for further study

19. Translation

20. Unexpected results

KEY IDEAS
Directions: Fill in the blanks or provide the appropriate responses.

1. To be useful, the evidence from data analysis needs to be:

2. When the results of the study are being interpreted, the researcher must use the following intellectual skills:

   a.

   b.

   c.

   d.

   e.

3. The initial evidence for the validity of the study results is derived from

   _____.

4. One of the assumptions often made in interpreting study results is that the study variables were

   _____.

5. Only the researcher knows how _____ the measures were taken.

6. List four questions that need to be asked regarding data analysis.

    a.

    b.

    c.

    d.

7. The value of evidence in any study is dependent on the

    _____ explained within the study.

8. Any report of nonsignificant results needs to indicate:

9. _____ are usually relationships found between variables that were not hypothesized and not predicted from the framework being used.

10. It is important to remember that research never _____.

11. What is one of the risks in developing conclusions in research?

12. Identify four characteristics of significant studies.

    a.

    b.

    c.

    d.

13. From the conservative perspective, one cannot generalize beyond

    _____.

14. Currently, nursing has few _____.

15. To formulate empirical generalizations, one must have evidence from

    _____.

16. Conclusions need to address applications to _____.

MAKING CONNECTIONS
Directions: Match each term with its definition.

Terms

a. Translate
b. Fidelity of data collection
c. Validation of qualitative analysis

d. Synthesis of findings
e. Interpret
f. Measures with poor validity and reliability

Definitions

_____ 1. Decision trail
_____ 2. Explain the meaning of information
_____ 3. Undetectable by computers
_____ 4. Use terms that can be more easily understood
_____ 5. Conclusions
_____ 6. Dependent on integrity of researcher

PUZZLES

Word Scramble
Directions: Unscramble the sentence below by rearranging the letters to form actual words. Note: You will use all the letters in every word.

Laveguatin het cherreas sproces duse ni eth dusty, cuprigdon gimeann morf teh strusle, nad torceginfas eth lusessfune fo teh dingfins, lal fo chiwh rae dinvlove ni treationinpert, errique gihh-veell tillteencula sporesecs.

Secret Message
Directions: Translate the secret message below by substituting one letter for another. For example, if you decide that "x" should really be "a," then "x" will be "a" every time it appears in this puzzle. Hint: Try to translate short words first to establish vowel patterns.

Oe vp qmpnqb, ojp pshrpctp nkea rxox xcxbmhm cpprm oe vp txkpnbbz

pwxahcpr, xchypr, xcr lhspc apxchcl, xcr veoj moxohmohtxb xcr tbhchtxb

mhlchnhtxctp cpprm oe vp pwxahcpr.

Crossword Puzzle

Directions: Complete the crossword puzzle below. Note: If the answer is more than one word, there are no blank spaces left between the words.

Across

3. Generate knowledge that influences a discipline.
7. Substantiation.
9. Synthesis and clarification of the meaning of study findings.
10. Change from one language to another.
11. Meaning of findings for clinical practice.

Down

1. Important information that is immediately useful.
2. Noteworthy.
4. Extending the conclusions beyond the sample.
5. Elucidation of study findings.
6. Interpreted results.
8. Products of research.

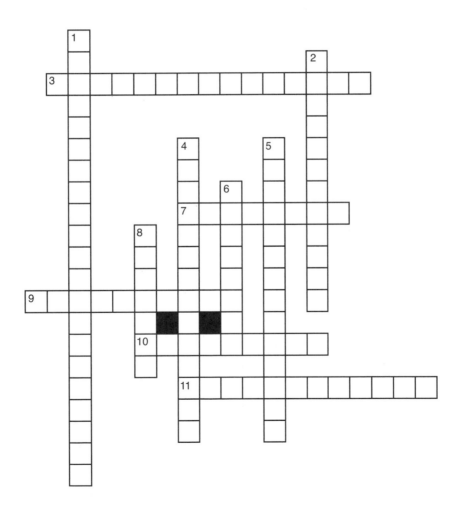

EXERCISES IN CRITIQUE

Directions: Review the Zalon (2004) study in Appendix B and answer the following questions. Consider the research question for Zalon's study: What is the relation of pain, depression, and fatigue to recovery, as measured by functional status and self-perception of recovery in older adults who have had major abdominal surgery?

1. Identify the findings reported by the author. Compare these findings to the results. Judge the appropriateness of the findings in relation to the results. Write a short evaluation of the linkage between the results and the findings.

2. Identify conclusions made by the author based on the findings.

3. Write a brief paragraph judging whether the conclusions are warranted by the data.

4. Identify the implications made by the author.

5. Write a brief paragraph evaluating the implications you identified in question 4. Include implications you were able to identify that were not considered by the author.

6. Write a brief paragraph assessing the clinical significance of the study's findings.

7. Were the findings generalized? If so, to what populations?

8. What suggestions did the author make for further studies?

GOING BEYOND

Using the questions above, perform a similar critique of the analyses used by Sethares and Elliott (2004).

CHAPTER 25

Communicating Research Findings

INTRODUCTION

Read Chapter 25 and then complete the following exercises. These exercises will assist you in understanding the process for developing the final research report and disseminating this report through presentations and publications to audiences of nurses, other health care professionals, policy makers, and health care consumers. The answers to these exercises are in Appendix A.

RELEVANT TERMS

Directions: Match each term with its correct definition.

Terms

a. Abstract
b. Communicating research findings
c. Duplicate publication

d. Poster session
e. Presentation
f. Publication

g. Query letter
h. Referred journal
i. Research report

Definitions

_____ 1. A visual presentation of a study using pictures, tables, and illustrations on a display board.

_____ 2. Developing a research report and disseminating it through presentations and publications to a variety of audiences.

_____ 3. A journal that uses expert reviewers to determine whether a manuscript is of acceptable quality for publication.

_____ 4. A letter sent to determine an editor's interest in reviewing a manuscript; it usually includes the research problem, a brief discussion of the major findings, the significance of the findings, and the researchers' qualifications for writing the article.

_____ 5. A clear, concise summary of a study that is usually limited to 100-250 words and briefly identifies the problem, purpose, framework, methodology, and results.

_____ 6. The practice of publishing the same article or major portions of the article in two or more print or electronic media without notifying the editors or referencing the other publications in the reference list.

_____ 7. Through this mechanism, research findings are permanently recorded in a journal or book.

_____ 8. Through this mechanism, research findings are verbally communicated at conferences and meetings.

_____   9. A document that provides a description of the research project and includes four major sections: introduction, methods, results, and discussion of the findings; this document is developed to promote communication of the research findings through presentation and publication.

KEY IDEAS

Directions: Fill in the blanks or provide the appropriate responses.

1. Identify four elements of the introduction section of a quantitative research report.

  a.

  b.

  c.

  d.

2. Identify the five content areas covered in the methods section of a quantitative research report.

  a.

  b.

  c.

  d.

  e.

3. A discussion of the level of significance (.05, .01, or .001) selected for a study is usually discussed in the _____ section of a research report.

4. The results section of a quantitative research report includes the

  _____ and the

  _____.

5. Nursing research reports sometimes use figures to provide a picture of the results. The commonly used figures in nursing research reports are _____ and

  _____.

6. The American Psychological Manual (APA, 1994) provides direction for the development of

   figures and tables used to display the _____ of a study.

7. The figures and tables in a research report _____ (*do* or *do not*) need to be referred to in the written text of the report.

8. The means and standard deviations for study variables should be included in the published

   study for use in future _____ and in conducting a _____ to determine sample size of future studies.

9. Nonsignificant findings are usually not presented in _____ and _____ but are discussed in the narrative of the research report.

10. Identify the five major content areas covered in the discussion section of a research report.

    a.

    b.

    c.

    d.

    e.

11. The theoretical importance of the study is determined by linking the study findings and conclu-

    sions to the study _____.

12. The discussion section has a link to practice by providing the

    _____.

13. The methods section of a qualitative research report includes a description of the researcher's role. What are the key parts of this role?

    a.

    b.

    c.

    d.

14. Identify the six elements that are usually covered in the introduction section of a qualitative research report.

    a.

    b.

    c.

    d.

    e.

    f.

15. The results of qualitative research might include the development of a _____ or

    _____, or the description of a _____, an historical _____,

    or a _____.

16. _____ and _____ are research reports that are developed in-depth by students as part of their requirements for a degree.

17. Nurses need to report their research findings to a variety of audiences, including:

    a.

    b.

    c.

    d.

18. More nurses need to be aware of research findings and their potential use for practice; therefore

    research reports need to be communicated to all nurses, including _____,

    _____, and _____.

19. The _____ electronic medium has greatly increased access to research findings as well as other health-related information.

20. Presenting research findings at a conference includes the following steps:

    a.

    b.

    c.

    d.

21. Acceptance as a presenter at most research conferences requires the submission of an

    _____.

22. An effective poster is a complete presentation of the study's contents, yet is easily comprehended in _____ minutes or less.

23. Advantage of a poster session is the opportunity for _____ interaction between the researcher and those viewing the poster.

24. Selecting a journal for publication of a study requires knowledge of the following:

    a.

    b.

    c.

25. *Nursing Research* journal editor prefers to receive a _____ regarding the possible publication of a manuscript.

26. Review of a manuscript by a potential publisher results in one of four possible decisions:

    a.

    b.

    c.

    d.

27. The most common reason manuscripts are rejected is that they are

    _____.

28. Complex qualitative studies might be published in _____ or in

    _____.

29. In a survey, 41 of 77 authors had published at least one form of duplicate article. Thus

    _____ is a serious concern in nursing literature.

30. Authors need to avoid unethical duplication by submitting original manuscripts or by providing full disclosure of any portion of a manuscript that has been previously published. Previous publications must be cited in the text of the manuscript and also in the

    _____.

MAKING CONNECTIONS

Directions: Match the sections of the quantitative research report listed below with the specific statements or elements from a research report.

Quantitative Research Report Sections

a. Introduction
b. Methods
c. Results
d. Discussion

Statements or Elements of a Research Report

_____   1.   This is a significant problem for nursing because the number of elderly is increasing, they are living longer, and they are experiencing more chronic illnesses and self-care deficits.

_____   2.   The sample was randomly selected from the seniors' Sunday school classes in four churches in a large metropolitan area.

_____   3.   The findings were supportive of the study framework.

_____   4.   The framework for the study was Orem's theory of self-care.

_____   5.   The data were analyzed using means, standard deviations, ranges, and analysis of variance to determine the differences among the three groups.

_____   6.   The purpose of the study was to examine the effects of a low intensity weight-lifting program on the muscle strength, balance, and performance of self-care behaviors in the elderly.

_____   7.   Tables and figures were used to present the results.

_____   8.   The limitations of the study were the small sample and the limited reliability and validity of the scale to measure self-care behaviors.

_____ 9. The quasi-experimental design of this study was an untreated control group design with pretest and posttest.

_____ 10. Future studies need to examine the impact of other interventions on the self-care and functional capacity of the elderly.

EXERCISES IN CRITIQUE

Sethares and Elliott Study

Directions: Review the Sethares and Elliott (2004) research article in Appendix B and answer the following questions.

1. Did the study include the major sections of a research report? Identify the sections of the research report.

2. Identify the audiences most likely to have read this journal article.

Wright Study

Directions: Review the Wright (2003) research article in Appendix B and answer the following questions.

1. Did the study include the major sections of a research report? Identify the sections of the research report.

2. Identify the audiences most likely to have read this journal article.

Zalon Study

Directions: Review the Zalon (2004) research article in Appendix B and answer the following questions.

1. Did the study include the major sections of a research report? Identify the sections of the research report.

2. Identify the audiences most likely to have read this journal article.

CHAPTER 26

Critical Analysis of Nursing Studies

INTRODUCTION

Read Chapter 26 and then complete the following exercises. These exercises will assist you in understanding the quantitative and qualitative research critique processes. The answers to these exercises are in Appendix A.

RELEVANT TERMS

Directions: Match each term with its correct definition.

Terms

a. Analysis step of critique
b. Analytic precision
c. Auditability
d. Comparison step of critique
e. Comprehension step of
f. Conceptual clustering
g. Context flexibility
h. Descriptive vividness
i. Evaluation step of critique
j. Heuristic relevance
k. Inductive reasoning skills
l. Intellectual critique of research
m. Methodological congruence
n. Theoretical connectedness
o. Transforming ideas across levels of abstraction

Definitions

_____ 1. Standard for evaluating qualitative research, in which documentation rigor, procedural rigor, ethical rigor, and auditability of the study are examined.

_____ 2. Rigorous development of a decision trail that is reported in sufficient detail to allow a second researcher to use the original data and the decision trail to arrive at conclusions similar to those of the original researcher.

_____ 3. Critique step that involves determining the strengths and limitations of the logical links connecting one study element with another.

_____ 4. Theoretical schema developed from a qualitative study; is clearly expressed, logically consistent, reflective of the data, and compatible with the knowledge base in nursing.

_____ 5. Critique step in which the ideal for each step of the quantitative research process is compared with the real steps in a published study.

_____ 6. Performing a series of transformations during which concrete data are transformed across several levels of abstractions to develop a theoretical schema that imparts meaning to the phenomenon under study.

_____ 7. Critique step during which the reader gains understanding of the terms in the research report; identifies the study elements; and grasps the nature, significance, and meaning of these elements.

_____ 8. Standard for evaluating a qualitative study in which the study's intuitive recognition, relationship to the existing body of knowledge, and applicability are examined.

_____ 9. Description of the site, subjects, experience of collecting data, and the researcher's thoughts during the qualitative research process presented clearly enough that the reader has the sense of personally experiencing the event.

_____ 10. A skill needed to critique qualitative studies that involves the capacity to switch from one context or world view to another, to shift perception in order to see things from a different perspective.

_____ 11. Involves a careful examination of all aspects of a study to judge the merits, limitations, meaning, and significance.

_____ 12. Last step of the critique process that involves the synthesis of study findings to determine the current body of knowledge in an area.

_____ 13. A skill needed to critique qualitative research that includes both deductive and inductive reasoning in order to follow the logic of the researcher.

_____ 14. Critique step in which the reader examines the meaning and significance of a study according to set criteria and compares it with previous studies conducted in the area.

_____ 15. A skill needed to critique qualitative research that involves moving from specific pieces of information and ideas to a synthesis of these ideas and a broader understanding of the phenomenon examined. An example of this skill is reviewing the literature, organizing the ideas from the review, and summarizing these ideas to determine the existing body of knowledge in a selected area.

KEY IDEAS
Directions: Fill in the blanks or provide the appropriate responses.

1. An intellectual research critique involves careful examination of all aspects of a study to judge

   the _____, _____, _____, and _____ of the study.

2. Identify three important questions that are part of an intellectual research critique.

   a.

   b.

   c.

3. Describe your role in conducting research critiques.

4. Identify four criteria that are usually addressed in critique of an abstract.

   a.

   b.

   c.

   d.

5. Conducting an intellectual critique of a quantitative study involves applying some basic guidelines that are outlined in your text. Identify three of these basic guidelines.

   a.

   b.

   c.

6. List the five steps of the quantitative research critique process.

   a.

   b.

   c.

   d.

   e.

7. Identify the five standards used to critique qualitative studies.

   a.

   b.

   c.

d.

e.

EXERCISES IN CRITIQUE

Directions: Read the research articles in Appendix B. Conduct critiques of these three studies using the guidelines in Chapter 26 in your text.

1. Conduct a critique of the Sethares and Elliott (2004) article using the guidelines outlined in your text. Many parts of this study were critiqued in Chapters 5 through 11 and Chapters 14-24 of this study guide.

   a. Conduct the comprehension step of the critique process. Questions are outlined in your text to direct your critique.

   b. Do a critique that includes the comparison, analysis, and evaluation steps of the quantitative research critique process.

2. Conduct a critique of the Wright (2003) article using the guidelines outlined in your text. Many parts of this study were critiqued in Chapters 4-9, 14-17, and 23 of this study guide.

   a. Conduct a critique of this study using the five standards of qualitative research: descriptive vividness, methodological congruence, analytical preciseness, theoretical connectedness, and heuristic relevance. Questions are outlined in your text to direct your critique.

3. Conduct a critique of the Zalon (2004) article using the guidelines outlined in your text. Many parts of this study were critiqued in Chapters 5-11 and Chapters 14-24 of this study guide.

   a. Conduct the comprehension step of the critique process. Questions are outlined in your text to direct your critique.

   b. Do a critique that includes the comparison, analysis, and evaluation steps of the quantitative research critique process.

CHAPTER 27

Using Research Knowledge to Promote an Evidence-Based Practice in Nursing

INTRODUCTION

Read Chapter 27 and then complete the following exercises. These exercises will assist you in understanding the process of using research findings in practice to develop and evidence-based practice for nursing. The answers to these exercises are in Appendix A.

RELEVANT TERMS

Directions: Match each term with its correct definition.

Terms

a. Adoption
b. Cognitive clustering
c. Communication of research findings
d. Conduct and Utilization of Research in Nursing (CURN) Project
e. Confirmation stage
f. Decision stage
g. Diffusion
h. Evidence-based practice
i. Evidence-based practice centers

j. Evidence-based practice guidelines
k. Grove Model for Implementing Evidence-Based Guidelines
l. Implementation stage
m. Innovation
n. Innovators
o. Iowa Model of Evidence-Based Practice
p. Knowledge stage

q. Meta-analysis
r. Persuasion stage
s. Research utilization
t. Rogers' innovation-decision process
u. Stetler's Model of Research Utilization
v. Western Interstate Commission for Higher Education (WICHE) Regional Nursing

Definitions

_____ 1. This involves the use of statistical analyses to merge the results from several completed studies to determine what is currently known and not known about a particular phenomenon.

_____ 2. Process that includes the steps of knowledge, persuasion, decision, implementation, and confirmation to promote diffusion or communication of research findings to members of a discipline.

_____ 3. Individuals who actively seek out new ideas and who are very effective in initiating the use of research findings in clinical practice.

_____   4.   Developing a research report and disseminating it through presentations and publications to practicing nurses, other health care professionals, policy makers, and consumers.

_____   5.   Idea, practice, or object that is perceived as new by an individual, a nursing unit, an entire agency, or other decision-making unit.

_____   6.   First major research utilization project in nursing that involved the collaboration of clinicians and educators in critiquing studies and developing detailed plans for using selected research findings in practice.

_____   7.   In Rogers' theory of diffusion, this stage occurs when the individual chooses to adopt or reject an innovation.

_____   8.   The purpose of this project was to increase the use of research findings in practice by communicating the findings, facilitating organizational modifications necessary for implementation, and encouraging collaborative research that is directly useful in clinical practice.

_____   9.   Patient care guidelines that are based on synthesized research findings from meta-analyses, integrative reviews of research, and extensive clinical trials; supported by consensus from recognized national experts; and affirmed by outcomes obtained by clinicians.

_____   10.   In Rogers' theory of diffusion, this stage occurs when an individual or group of individuals form an attitude toward an innovation.

_____   11.   In Rogers' theory of diffusion, this is the stage when the first awareness of the existence of the innovation occurs.

_____   12.   This is a comprehensive framework to enhance the use of research findings by nurses that includes the phases of preparation, validation, comparative evaluation/decision making, translation/application, and evaluation.

_____   13.   Model developed by one of the textbook authors to promote the use of evidence-based guidelines in practice.

_____   14.   Centers designated by the Agency for Healthcare Research and Quality for the development or research in designated areas and the translation of the evidence-based research findings into clinical practice.

_____   15.   The process by which an innovation is communicated through certain channels over time among the members of a social system.

_____   16.   This process involves the full acceptance of an innovation and the implementation of the ideas in practice.

_____   17.   The process of synthesizing, disseminating, and using research-generated knowledge to make an impact on or a change in the existing practices in society.

_____   18.   In Rogers' theory of diffusion, this stage occurs when an individual or agency evaluates the effectiveness of the innovation and decides to continue or discontinue it.

_____   19.   A model developed by Titler and colleagues in 1994 and revised in 2001 that provides direction for the development of evidence-based practice in a clinical agency.

_____   20.   In Rogers' theory of diffusion, this stage occurs when an individual or agency uses an innovation.

_____ 21.   The integration and synthesis of findings from scientifically sound research.

_____ 22.   A practice that involves the conscientious integration of best research evidence with clinical expertise and patient values and needs in the delivery of quality, cost-effective health care.

KEY IDEAS

Directions: Fill in the blanks or provide the appropriate responses.

1. List three reasons nursing needs to develop an evidence-based practice.

   a.

   b.

   c.

2. What utilization theory was used in nursing but was not developed by a nurse?

3. Identify three sources you might access to keep current with the research literature.

   a.

   b.

   c.

4. Identify two reports published as a result of the WICHE project.

   a.

   b.

5. Identify the four-step research utilization process used in the CURN project.

   a.

   b.

   c.

   d.

6. Identify three prior conditions of an agency that need to be examined when planning to make a change based on research.

a.

b.

c.

7. Identify three areas where research findings were considered worthy of implementation in practice in the CURN project.

a.

b.

c.

8. Identify the three types of barriers to using research findings in nursing practice and provide an example of each.

a.

Example:

b.

Example:

c.

Example:

9. Identify the five characteristics of an innovation or change in practice to examine during the persuasion stage of Rogers' Utilization Model.

a.

b

c.

d.

e.

10. Active rejection of a change in practice involves:

11. Passive rejection of a change in practice indicates:

12. Identify and describe three ways that research findings might be implemented in nursing practice that were discussed in Stetler's Model of Research Utilization to facilitate evidence-based practice.

a.

Description:

b.

Description:

c.

Description:

13. During Rogers' confirmation stage, discontinuance of the change in practice can occur. What are the two types of discontinuance?

a.

b.

14. Identify two sources of summaries of nursing research knowledge.

a.

b.

15. Identify the five phases of the Stetler Model of Research Utilization.

    a.

    b.

    c.

    d.

    e.

16. The comparative evaluation phase of Stetler's Model includes four parts: substantiating evidence, fit of the setting, _____, and _____.

17. Identify the three options of the decision-making phase of the Stetler's Model.

    a.

    b.

    c.

18. The _____ Model was developed in 1994 and revised in 2001 to promote evidence-based practice in nursing.

19. The Joint National Committee on Prevention, Detection, Evaluation, and Treatment of High Blood Pressure (JNC VVII) guideline that was published in 2003 is an example of

    _____.

20. The goal of the Grove Model for Implementing Evidence-Based Guidelines is

    _____.

MAKING CONNECTIONS

Directions: Match the stage in Rogers' research utilization process with the appropriate description and/or example.

Stages

a. Knowledge
b. Persuasion
c. Decision

d. Implementation
e. Confirmation

Descriptions

_____ 1. The stage when nurses evaluate the cost-effectiveness and the impact on quality of care of using the Braden scale to prevent pressure ulcers in hospitalized patients.

_____ 2. The stage when nurses reject a protocol for treatment of stage IV pressure ulcers in the elderly.

_____ 3. The first awareness of the existence of an exercise program for severely disabled children obtained from attending a research conference and reading the study in a research journal.

_____ 4. Research knowledge about the exercise program was directly used in the nursing practice of a rehabilitation center.

_____ 5. Nurses held groups to discuss the pros and cons of using new ideas in practice.

Directions: Match the type of adopter from Rogers' research utilization theory with the appropriate description and/or example.

Types of Adopters

a. Early adopters
b. Early majority
c. Innovators

d. Laggards
e. Late majority

Descriptions

_____ 1. These individuals are either the last to adopt a new idea or never adopt the idea. They are often security-oriented, tend to cling to the past, and isolated in a system.

_____ 2. Clinical specialists, nurse practitioners, and in-services educators are often referred to as this type of adopter.

_____ 3. These individuals are skeptical about new ideas and will adopt them only if group pressure is great.

_____ 4. These individuals have a high level of mass media exposure and interpersonal networks that are widely extended, reaching beyond their local social system. They comprise only 2.5% of the adopters.

_____   5. These individuals are rarely leaders but are active followers and will readily follow in the use of a new idea.

GOING BEYOND

1. Answer the following questions about the clinical agency where you are currently doing your clinical hours:

   a. Are the agency's policies and nursing protocols and algorithms based on research?

   b. What is the basis of the policies and protocols, if not research?

   c. Who are the innovators in this agency? (Identify them by their positions.)

   d. Who might be resistant to change?

   e. Does the agency provide research publications for nurses? Provide some examples of these publications.

   f. Does the agency have the goal of evidence-based practice?

   g. Is the agency seeking magnet status?

2. Conduct a project to promote evidence-based practice in a selected area of your practice. Use the following steps as a guide:

   a. Identify a clinical problem that might be improved by using research knowledge.

   b. Locate and review the studies in this problem area. (A list of integrated reviews of research and meta-analyses is provided on the textbook website.)

   c. Summarize what is known and not known regarding this problem.

   d. Select a model or theory to direct your use of research findings in practice, such as Rogers' theory of utilization, Stetler's Model of Research Utilization to facilitate evidence-based practice, or Iowa Model of Evidence-Based Practice.

   e. Assess your agency's readiness to make the change.

   f. Communicate the evidence-based change proposed to the nursing personnel, other health professionals, and administration.

   g. Support those persons involved in making the evidence-based change in practice.

h. Implement the evidence-based change by developing a protocol, algorithm, or policy to be used in practice.

i. Develop evaluation strategies to determine the effect of the evidence-based change on patient, provider, and agency outcomes.

j. Evaluate overtime to determine whether the evidence-based change should be continued. You might also extend the change to additional units or clinical agencies.

3. Use the Grove Model for Implementing Evidence-Based Guidelines to implement an evidence-based guideline from the Agency for Healthcare Research and Quality website in your practice.

CHAPTER 28

Proposal Writing for Research Approval

INTRODUCTION

Read Chapter 28 and then complete the following exercises. These exercises will assist you in understanding the process of writing a research proposal and receiving approval to conduct the study. The answers to these exercises are in Appendix A.

RELEVANT TERMS

Directions: Match each term with its definition.

Terms

a. Approval process
b. Condensed proposal
c. Preproposal

d. Research proposal
e. Verbal defense of a proposal

Definitions

_____ 1. A written plan identifying the major elements of a study, such as problem, purpose, and framework, and outlining the methods to conduct the study; a formal way to communicate ideas about a proposed study, to receive approval to conduct the study, and to seek funding.

_____ 2. Presentation and clarification of the proposed research project to the members of the agency's institutional review board.

_____ 3. A short document (4-5 pages plus appendixes) written to explore the funding possibilities for a research project.

_____ 4. A process implemented by a researcher to obtain permission to conduct a study in a selected agency.

_____ 5. A proposal of limited length that is developed for review by clinical agencies and funding institutions.

KEY IDEAS

Directions: Fill in the blanks or provide the appropriate responses.

1. A quality proposal is clear, _____, and _____.

2. Writing a quality proposal involves:

  a.

  b.

  c.

  d.

3. A commonly used format in developing a nursing research proposal is the

  _____ (_____) format.

4. A quantitative research proposal usually includes the following sections:

  a.

  b.

  c.

  d.

5. Presenting a design for quasi-experimental and experimental studies involves:

  a.

  b.

  c.

  d.

  e.

  f.

  g.

6. Conducting research in a clinical agency requires approval by the

  _____ board (_____).

7. Identify at least four content areas covered in the introduction section of a qualitative research proposal.

   a.

   b.

   c.

   d.

8. A preproposal includes:

   a.

   b.

   c.

   d.

   e.

9. Clinical agencies and health care corporations review studies for the following reasons:

   a.

   b.

   c.

10. As part of the approval process, the researcher must determine the agency's policy regarding:

   a.

   b.

   c.

11. If a study is funded, changes in a study must be discussed with the _____ of

   the _____.

12. List the questions that a researcher needs to address before revising a research project.

a.

b.

c.

MAKING CONNECTIONS

Directions: Match the processes listed below with the steps that follow.

Processes

a. Proposal development process
b. Approval process for research

Steps

_____   1. Requires developing an esthetically appealing copy.

_____   2. Involves examining the impact of conducting the study on the reviewing institution.

_____   3. Includes an introduction, review of relevant literature, framework, and methods and procedures sections.

_____   4. Involves examining the social and political factors in an agency where the study is to be conducted.

_____   5. Includes a verbal defense of the proposed study to the institutional review board (IRB) of the agency.

GOING BEYOND

1. Identify a significant nursing problem and develop a research proposal to direct the investigation of this problem. Use the guidelines in Chapter 28 of your text as a basis for developing the proposal and seek the assistance or your instructor in revising and formulating the final proposal.

2. Identify an agency where your proposed study might be conducted. Seek approval from that agency to conduct your study.

CHAPTER 29

Seeking Funding for Research

INTRODUCTION

Read Chapter 29 and then complete the following exercises. These exercises will assist you in learning relevant terms and understanding the process of seeking funding for research. The answers to these exercises are in Appendix A.

RELEVANT TERMS

Directions: Define the following terms in your own words without looking at your textbook. Then check your definitions with those in the glossary of your textbook. Using this strategy, you can identify elements of the term that are not yet clear in your mind. Reread the relevant section of the chapter to clarify your understanding of the term.

1. Developmental grant

2. Funded research

3. Grantsmanship

4. Foundation grant

5. Networking

6. Mentor

7. Pink sheet

8. Query letter

9. Reference group

10. Requests for applications (RFA)

11. Requests for proposals (RFP)

12. Research grant

13. Researcher-initiated proposal

233

KEY IDEAS

Directions: Fill in the blanks or provide the appropriate responses.

1. As the control of variance and the complexity of the design increase,

   _____.

2. _____ and funding for research are interrelated.

3. _____ may be stepping stones to larger grants.

4. Funding agencies are usually more supportive of researchers who do what?

5. An aspiring researcher needs to _____
   in a specific area of study.

6. What can help researchers become better able to critique their own proposals and revise them?

7. _____ often provide the first step in being recognized as a credible researcher.

8. The book most useful in determining funding available from foundations is the

   _____.

9. In preparing a proposal to a foundation, the _____ need to be
   followed carefully.

10. The largest source of grant monies is _____.

11. The most complete source of information on federal funding sources is the

    _____.

12. If a researcher is preparing a researcher-initiated proposal for federal funding, it is useful to:

13. RFPs are published in the _____.

14. Because a number of researchers will be responding to the same RFP and only one or a few

    proposals will be approved, these proposals are considered _____.

15. An RFA is similar to an RFP except that with the RFA, the government agency

_____ .

16. After submission, a federal proposal is assigned to _____ for scientific evaluation.

17. Receipt of money to initiate a federal grant may not occur for up to _____ after submission of the proposal.

18. Seeking funding for a second grant needs to be initiated

_____ .

MAKING CONNECTIONS

1. List four strategies that can be used to gain skills in grantsmanship.

a.

b.

c.

d.

2. List four sources of small grant funding.

a.

b.

c.

d.

PUZZLES

Word Scramble

Directions: Unscramble the sentence below by rearranging the letters to form actual words. Note: You will use all the letters in every word.

Lewl-geseddin dusties nac eb sexpivene.

Secret Message

Directions: Translate the secret message below by substituting one letter for another. For example, if you decide that "x" should really be "t," then "x" will be "t" every time it appears in this puzzle. Hint: Try to translate short words first to establish vowel patterns.

Xfi ukeizxehek kvijelebexo yh xfi xvyhiuueyz eu vibmtij xy xfi wsmblxo yh

uxsjeiu kyzjskxij lo exu viuimvkfivu.

Crossword Puzzle

Directions: Complete the crossword puzzle on the next page. Note: If the answer is more than one word, there are no blank spaces left between the words.

Across

1. Grant-supported study.
6. Form sent from government agency rejecting and critiquing a proposal.
8. Adviser.
9. Request for proposals on government-identified topic.
10. Skill in writing proposals.
11. Funded study.
12. Proposal to fulfill government contract.

Down

2. A number of people with common interests and aspirations.
3. Connection with researchers who have common interests.
4. Funding by a private agency.
5. Proposal to implement a new program.
7. Inquiry about the interest of a journal in publishing an article.

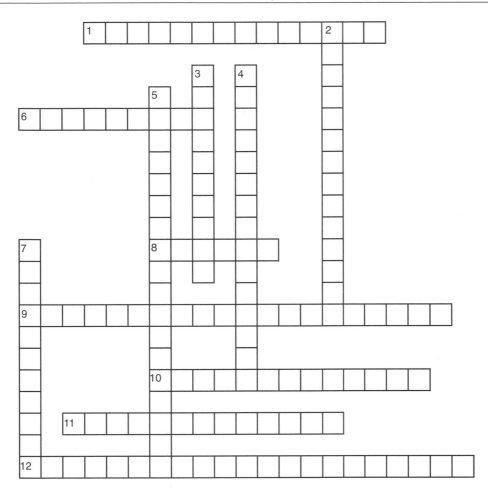

GOING BEYOND

1. Ask a faculty member for permission to read a research proposal for which he or she has received funding.

2. Ask a faculty member for permission to read a research proposal that was not funded and the associated pink sheet.

Answers

CHAPTER 1

Relevant Terms

1. k	8. s	14. a
2. m	9. j	15. g
3. b	10. q	16. i
4. h	11. r	17. e
5. p	12. c	18. l
6. n	13. f	19. o
7. d		

Key Ideas

1. Description involves identifying the nature and attributes of nursing phenomena. Descriptive knowledge generated through research can be used to identify what exists in nursing practice, discover new information, and classify information of use in the discipline (for example, description of those who are at risk for HIV or description of the trends of obesity in society).

2. Explanation focuses on clarifying relationships among variables or identifying reasons why certain events occur. For example, risk of developing pressure ulcers is related to level of mobility and age; as mobility decreases and age increases, pressure ulcer risk increases.

3. Prediction involves estimating the probability of a specific outcome in a given situation. With predictive knowledge, nurses can anticipate the effects certain nursing interventions might have on patients and families (for example, predicting the effects of an exercise program in the schools on children's weight).

4. Control is the ability to manipulate a situation to produce the desired outcome. Thus nurses could develop and implement certain interventions to help patients and families achieve quality outcomes (for example, the use of warm, *not cold*, applications for the resolution of normal IV infiltrations; or diet and exercise to promote weight loss).

Making Connections

1. You could have identified any of the following ways of acquiring knowledge in nursing. Some possible examples of each way of acquiring nursing knowledge are provided.
   a. Tradition: giving patients a bath everyday in the morning.
   b. Authority: expert clinical nurses, educators, and authors of articles or books.
   c. Borrowing: using knowledge from medicine or psychology to provide nursing care.
   d. Trial and error: trying a particular position to help a patient reduce her discomfort during labor.
   e. Personal experience: obtaining knowledge by being in a clinical agency and providing care to patients and families.
   f. Role modeling: a new graduate in an internship is mentored by an expert nurse who role-models quality nursing care behaviors for the new graduate.
   g. Intuition: knowing that a patient's condition is deteriorating but having no concrete data to support this feeling or hunch.

h. Reasoning: reasoning from the general to the specific (deductive reasoning); reasoning from the specific to the general (inductive reasoning).
i. Research: quantitative and qualitative research methods.
2. Personal experience
3. Novice, advanced beginner, competent, proficient, and expert
4. Borrowed
5. Research or empirical
6. Intuition
7. Traditions
8. Mentors
9. Role models
10. Inductive and deductive
11. Deductive reasoning
12. Use the content in your textbook on Acquiring Knowledge in Nursing to determine the knowledge base for each of the interventions you identified. Nursing knowledge is acquired through tradition, authority, borrowing, trial and error, personal experience, role modeling, intuition, reasoning, and research.
13. You need to examine the interventions you use in clinical practice and decide which way of acquiring knowledge you use most frequently: tradition, authority, borrowing, trial and error, personal experience, role modeling, intuition, reasoning, or research. It is important to increase the use of research evidence in the implementation of interventions in practice.
14. American Nurses Association (2003) identified the following areas of focus for nursing knowledge: promotion of health and safety; care and self-care processes; physical, emotional, and spiritual comfort, discomfort, and pain; adaptation to physiologic and pathophysiologic processes; emotions related to experiences of birth, growth and development, health, illness, disease, and death; meanings ascribed to health and illness; decision making and ability to make choices; relationships, role performance,

and change processes within relationships; social policies and their effects on the health of individuals, families, and communities; health care systems and their relationships with access to and quality of health care; and the environment and the prevention of disease (Burns & Grove, 2005, p. 12).
15. The types of research conducted in nursing include quantitative, qualitative, outcomes, and intervention research.
16. A variety of philosophical beliefs could be identified, including holistic perspective in providing health care, importance of the family in caring for a patient, providing access to care for patients regardless of their financial status, and providing physical, emotional, and social care to patient and family.
17. Evidence-based practice

Puzzles

Nursing research is directly linked to these concepts: theory, empirical world (nursing practice), science, and abstract thought processes. There are indirect links of nursing research to philosophy, knowledge, and ways of knowing.

Word Scramble

Nursing research is directly linked to the world of nursing.

CHAPTER 2

Relevant Terms

1. i	8. r	14. g
2. c	9. a	15. l
3. e	10. f	16. d
4. k	11. n	17. b
5. q	12. s	18. j
6. o	13. p	19. h
7. m		

Key Ideas

1. Nightingale

2. 1952
3. ANA Council of Nurse Researchers
4. Research
5. *Research in Nursing & Health*
6. *Western Journal of Nursing Research*
7. *Scholarly Inquiry for Nursing Practice, Applied Nursing Research, Nursing Science Quarterly*
8. Conduct and Utilization of Research in Nursing (CURN)
9. Summaries of current research knowledge in the areas of nursing practice, nursing care delivery, nursing education, and the profession of nursing
10. 1985
11. National Institute for Nursing Research (NINR)
12. Conduct, support, and dissemination
13. You could have identified any of the following research priorities or themes for NINR:
    a. Changing lifestyle behaviors for better health
    b. Managing the effects of chronic illness to improve quality of life
    c. Identifying effective strategies to reduce health disparities
    d. Harnessing advanced technologies to serve human needs
    e. Enhancing the end-of-life experience for patients and their families
14. Clinical and/or outcomes research
15. Professional Standards Review Organizations (PSROs)
16. Agency for Health Care Policy and Research (AHCPR)
17. Evidence-based
18. Agency for Healthcare Research and Quality (AHRQ)
19. The goals of AHRQ are:
    a. Support improvements in health outcomes
    b. Strengthen quality measurements and improvements
    c. Identify strategies to improve access, foster appropriate use of health care

resources, and reduce unnecessary expenditures
20. Focus of *Healthy People 2010* is health promotion and illness prevention.

Making Connections

Processes

1. a	5. b
2. c	6. a
3. a	7. c
4. c	8. c

Research Methods

1. b	5. a	8. a
2. b	6. a	9. b
3. a	7. a	10. a
4. b		

Nurses' Educational Preparation

1. a	5. b
2. e	6. c
3. b	7. d or e
4. d	

Puzzles

Word Scramble

Both quantitative and qualitative research methods are essential to nursing knowledge. Research knowledge is needed to control outcomes in nursing practice.

Exercises in Critique

Research Types

1. b
2. a
3. b

Expertise of the Researchers in the Critique Studies

Research, educational, and clinical expertise of the authors for the three critique articles are described. Answers for these questions are found on the front page of each of the three articles in the section that addresses the education and positions of the authors and the funding for the studies.

1. Sethares is a registered nurse with a doctorate in philosophy (PhD). A PhD is a research degree, indicating this author has conducted previous research. Elliott is a master's-prepared registered nurse and a certified adult nurse practitioner (ANP-C). To be certified as an ANP, Elliott must be currently involved in clinical practice. Funding was obtained for this study from the University of Massachusetts Dartmouth Foundation, indicating it was reviewed by the University and approved for funding. university review of research involves extensive examination of the quality of the study and the expertise of the researchers proposing it.

2. Wright has a PhD, which indicates her educational preparation as a researcher. She works on the National Institutes for Health (NIH) Stroke Neuroscience Unit. NIH is a national research funding agency within the federal government. This neuroscience unit is a research unit and indicates that Wright is both a strong researcher and clinician.

3. Zalon is a registered nurse (RN) and doctorally (PhD) prepared, indicating she has educational preparation for conducting this study. In addition, she is an advanced practice registered nurse (APRN) who is board-certified (BC). These credentials indicate that Zalon is currently involved in clinical practice and has certification in her area of specialization. This study was funded by the National Institute of Nursing Research and an internal faculty research grant from the University of Scranton. Thus both the university and the federal funding agency reviewed the proposal for this study and examined the qualifications of the researcher. Their funding of this study indicates that they determined the study was of quality and the researcher had the expertise to conduct the study. The information on funding for this study is found prior to the list of references.

CHAPTER 3

Relevant Terms

1. s	11. k	20. n
2. z	12. i	21. l
3. a	13. u	22. d
4. e	14. b	23. aa
5. y	15. h	24. f
6. c	16. t	25. o
7. p	17. v	26. m
8. w	18. bb	27. g
9. q	19. x	28. j
10. r		

Key Ideas

Control in Quantitative Research

1. Highly controlled
2. Quasi-experimental and experimental
3. Descriptive or correlational
4. Experimental
5. Nonrandom; random
6. Natural
7. Highly controlled
8. Experimental
9. Partially controlled
10. Quasi-experimental

Steps of the Research Process

1. Problem-solving process; nursing process
2. Problem; purpose
3. Methodology
4. Outcomes; communication of findings; use of findings in practice
5. Step 1: Research problem and purpose
   Step 2: Literature review
   Step 3: Study framework
   Step 4: Research objectives, questions, or hypotheses
   Step 5: Study variables
   Step 6: Assumptions
   Step 7: Limitations

Step 8: Research design
Step 9: Population and sample
Step 10: Methods of measurement
Step 11: Data collection
Step 12: Data analysis
Step 13: Research outcomes

6. Assumptions are statements taken for granted or considered true even though they have not been scientifically tested.

7. You could identify any of the following assumptions (Williams, 1980, p. 48):
   a. People want to assume control of their own health problems.
   b. Stress should be avoided.
   c. People are aware of the experiences that most affect their life choices.
   d. Health is a priority for most people.
   e. People in underserved areas feel underserved.
   f. Most measurable attitudes are held strongly enough to direct behavior.
   g. Health professionals view health care in a different manner than do laypersons.
   h. Human biological and chemical factors show less variation than do cultural and social factors.
   i. The nursing process is the best way of conceptualizing nursing practice.
   j. Statistically significant differences relate to the variable or variables under consideration.
   k. People operate on the basis of cognitive information.
   l. Increased knowledge about an event lowers anxiety about the event.
   m. Receipt of health care at home is preferable to receipt of care in an institution.

8. Study limitations are theoretical and methodological restrictions or weaknesses in a study that may decrease the generalizability of the findings.

9. Limitations include such factors as a nonrepresentative sample, small sample size, weak design with threats to design validity, single setting, instruments with limited reliability and validity, limited control over data collection, weak implementation of the treatment, and improper use of statistical analyses.

10. Pilot study

11. You could identify any of the following reasons for conducting a pilot study:
    a. To determine whether the proposed study is feasible (e.g., Are the subjects available? Does the researcher have the time and money to do the study?)
    b. To develop or refine a research treatment
    c. To develop a protocol for the implementation of a treatment
    d. To identify problems with the design
    e. To determine whether the sample is representative of the population or whether the sampling technique is effective
    f. To examine the reliability and validity of the research instruments
    g. To develop or refine data collection instruments
    h. To refine the data collection and analysis plan
    i. To give the researcher experience with the subjects, setting, methodology, and methods of measurement
    j. To try out data analysis techniques

Making Connections

Types of Quantitative Research

1. c	7. a	13. c
2. a	8. b	14. a
3. b	9. c	15. c
4. a	10. d	16. a
5. c	11. b	17. c
6. d	12. a	

Puzzles

Word Scramble

Quantitative research methods include descriptive, correlational, quasi-experimental, and experimental studies.

Crossword Puzzle

Across

2. Design
4. Quantitative
8. Problem
9. Hypothesis
10. Basic
12. Measurement
14. Framework
16. Setting
17. Rigor
18. Sample
19. Question

Down

1. Outcome
2. Data
3. Study
5. Assumptions
6. Variable
7. Literature
11. Control
13. Process
15. Applied

Exercises in Critique

1. c. Sethares and Elliott (2004) conducted a quasi-experimental study with a treatment for patients with heart failure.
2. e. Wright (2003) conducted a phenomenological qualitative study of recovery from substance abuse.
3. b. Zalon (2004) conducted a correlational study of elderly recovering from abdominal surgery.
4. a. Applied quantitative study
5. a. Applied qualitative study
6. a. Applied quantitative study

Going Beyond

Develop two ideas for quantitative studies and have your faculty review and discuss them with you. The section on making connections includes several ideas for quantitative studies.

CHAPTER 4

Relevant Terms

Check the glossary in the back of your text for definitions.

Key Ideas

1. Discovering meanings
2. Perceptually putting pieces together to make wholes

3. Get outside of any existing theories or gestalts that explain the phenomenon of interest
4. A particular philosophical stance thought to be a paradigm
5. Openness, scrupulous adherence to a philosophical perspective thoroughness in collecting data, and consideration of all of the data in the subjective theory development phase
6. Describe experiences as they are lived, to capture the lived experience of study participants
7. People define reality and how their beliefs are related to their actions
8. Created by people through attaching meanings to situations
9. Portrait of a people
10. Describe a culture through examining various cultural characteristics
11. Where have we come from, who are we, where are we going?
12. The structure of a science and the process of thinking about and valuing certain phenomena held in common by the science
13. Principles to guide conduct based on ethical theories
14. Uncover the distortions and constraints that impede free, equal, and uncoerced participation in society

Making Connections

1. Characteristics of rigor in qualitative research:
   a. Openness
   b. Scrupulous adherence to a philosophical perspective
   c. Thoroughness in collecting data
   d. Consideration of all of the data in the subjective theory development phase

Qualitative Methods

1. c
2. b
3. a
4. c

5. a
6. d
7. c
8. b
9. d
10. a

Puzzles

Crossword Puzzle

Across	**Down**
1. Emergent fit	2. Foundations
3. Ethnonursing	4. Culture
5. Deconstruct	9. Reconstructing
6. Material	11. Philosophical
7. Participatory	12. Intervention
8. Grounded	13. Ethnographic
10. Rigor	15. Cognitive
14. Ethics	17. Context
16. Phenomenological	19. Discovery
18. Being	
20. Ethnoscientific	
21. Descriptive	
22. Sedimented	
23. Embodied	
24. Situated	

Word Scramble

Once you have ascended to the open context, you cannot go back to the idea that the phenomenon you have observed can be seen only one way.

Secret Message

It is critical to understand the philosophy on which each qualitative method is based. (Do you know your Greek letters?)

Exercises in Critique

1. Phenomenology
2. Because ascending to an open construct is internal, one can only judge by the author's comments. The journaling used by the author would facilitate this process.
3. Giorgi's method

4. Bracketing (journaling)
   Discussion of recorded interviews with senior researchers
   Presenting data from naive units to clustering to themes to essential descriptions

CHAPTER 5

Relevant Terms

1. b	5. f	8. j
2. h	6. i	9. d
3. g	7. c	10. e
4. a		

Key Ideas

Research Problem and Purpose

1. a. Variables
   b. Population
   c. Setting
2. Any of the following responses might be given:
   a. Has an impact on nursing practice
   b. Builds on previous research
   c. Used to develop evidence-based practice
   d. Promotes theory development
   e. Promotes theory testing
   f. Addresses current concerns or priorities in nursing and health care
3. Landmark; Agency for Healthcare Research and Quality (AHRQ)
4. Replicated
5. Approximate or operational
6. a. Researchers' expertise
   b. Money commitment
   c. Availability of subjects, facility, and equipment
   d. Study's ethical considerations
7. Educational preparation, conduct of previous research, and clinical experience in nursing practice.
8. The common sources of research problems include, but are not limited to, the following:
   a. Nursing practice

b. Researcher and peer interactions

c. Literature review: replicating previous studies, using study ideas generated by previous researchers, and identifying gaps in the knowledge base of a selected research topic

d. Theoretical propositions or relationships expressed in theories

e. Research priorities identified by funding agencies and specialty groups and organizations

9. The priority goals of outcomes research include the following, but other goals might be listed that would improve the outcomes for patients and families, providers, and health care agencies.

a. Avoid adverse effects of care

b. Improve the patient's physiologic, mental, and social status

c. Reduce the patient's signs and symptoms

d. Improve the patient's functional status and well-being

e. Achieve patient satisfaction

f. Minimize the cost of care

g. Maximize revenues of care

h. Improve access to care

i. Improve quality of care delivered by providers

j. Improve the quality of care provided by health care agencies

10. Research topics

11. Research purposes

Making Connections

1. g	6. j	11. h
2. c	7. e	12. a
3. h	8. i	13. j
4. f	9. d	14. g
5. a	10. c	

Exercises in Critique

Sethares and Elliott (2004) Study

1. a. Problem significance: "Cardiovascular disease, the leading cause of health in the United States today, is one of the most prevalent chronic illnesses of adulthood. A common clinical endpoint of many cardiovascular disorders if heart failure (HF) . . . The American College of Cardiology/American Heart Association Task Force reports that 4.8 million Americans experience HF, with 550,000 new cases and 50,000 deaths reported annually. In 1999, 962,000 Americans were discharged from acute care facilities with a primary diagnosis of HF, the most prevalent diagnosis in those aged more than 65 year" (Sethares & Elliott, 2004, p. 249).

b. Background of the problem: "HF is characterized by an unstable course of illness with unpredictable exacerbations and progression of symptoms, often without further damage to the myocardium . . . Because HF is a chronic condition, most lifestyle change is made on an outpatient basis, necessitating follow-up in the home setting to evaluate medication effectiveness, monitor symptoms, and promote self-care behaviors. However, current capitation rates fiscally limit the quality of nursing care provided in the home" (Sethares & Elliott, 2004, p. 249).

c. Problem statement: "It is imperative that nurses develop innovative methods to improve the self-care behaviors of this population while attempting to decrease costly rehospitalizations. A tailored message intervention is one proposed alternative" (Sethares & Elliott, 2004, p. 249).

2. Study purpose: The purpose of this study is to "determine the efficacy of a tailored message intervention administered during hospital admission and at 1 week and 1 month after discharge on HF readmission rates, reported quality of life, and perceived benefit and barrier beliefs in elderly patients with HF" (Sethares & Elliott, 2004, p. 251).

3. The problem and purpose are significant since a large number of adults are affected by HF and this is such a costly chronic illness. Nurses are uniquely positioned to education patients and assist them in coping with chronic illnesses such as HF. More research is needed to find more effect interventions to assist patients with HF.

4. Yes, the variables, population, and settings are identified in the study purpose.
   a. Independent variable is tailored message intervention, and the dependent variables are HF readmission rates, reported quality of life, and perceived benefit and barrier beliefs. Thus the study had 1 intervention and 4 outcome variables.
   b. Population: Elderly patients with HF
   c. Settings: Both hospital and homes of patients

5. The problem and purpose are feasible because (1) the study was funded by a grant from the University of Massachusetts Dartmouth Foundation; (2) researchers had research and clinical expertise, as discussed in Chapter 2 of this study guide; (3) adequate subjects were available to participate in the study; (4) hospital personnel were supportive of the study; (5) no special equipment was needed for the study; and (6) the study was ethical and protected the rights of the subjects.

Wright (2003) Study

1. a. "Recovery from substance abuse is a recovery phenomenon that is of importance to nursing. Reports in the literature indicate that recovery from substance abuse is a complex multidimensional process that occurs both with and without expert assistance . . . The recidivism rate for substance abusers has been reported to be at 90% 12 months after treatment, with most relapses occurring after 3 months" (Wright, 2003, p. 173).
   b. Background of the problem: "For many

African American women recovering from substance abuse, current treatment modalities, and self-help groups do not meet their needs (Hooks, 1993; Nelson-Zlupko, Dore, Kauffman, & Kaltenbach, 1996), because mainstream treatment of substance abuse has traditionally been developed and implemented by male providers for male clients (Abbott, 1994; Reed, 1985) . . . Research suggests that women may benefit from substance abuse programs that include a residential component, as well as gender-specific services (Dempsey & Wenner, 1996; Nelson-Zlupko, et al., 1996). Spirituality has often been noted in the health care literature to affect recovery (Ellison & Levin, 1998; McNichol, 1996; Sloan, Bagiella, & Powell, 1999)" (Wright, 2003, pp. 173-174).
   c. Problem statement: "A phenomenological understanding of all that spirituality may represent to African American women is relevant to the recovery process from substance abuse" (Wright, 2003, p. 174).

2. Study purpose: "A qualitative phenomenological research study was designed to explore the essential elements of the lived experience of spirituality among African American women recovering from substance abuse and to describe the meanings made of this phenomenon by the person experiencing it" (Wright, 2003, p. 174).

3. The problem and purpose are significant since they focus on a common problem of substance abuse that is complex and requires extensive understanding and a variety of strategies to treat. In addition, limited research has been done to facilitate understanding of women and substance abuse treatment and the impact of spirituality on the recovery process. Wright (2003) clearly indicates the problem is significant to nursing and encourages nurses to increase their involvement in recognizing and treating

African American women with substance abuse problems.

4. The research concept and population are identified, but not the setting in the study purpose.
   a. Research concept is the lived experience of spirituality in recovery from substance abuse.
   b. Population: African American women recovering from substance abuse
   c. Setting: Not identified in the study purpose

5. The problem and purpose are feasible because (1) the study was conducted on a National Institute of Health (NIH) Unit; (2) researcher had research and clinical expertise, as discussed in Chapter 2 of this study guide; (3) adequate subjects were available to participate in the study; (4) NIH personnel were supportive of this study; (5) no special equipment was needed for the study; and (6) the study was ethical and protected the rights of the subjects.

Zalon (2004) Study

1. a. Significance of the problem: "The leading complication of hospitalization for older patients is functional decline, which is associated with longer hospital stays, increased mortality, higher rates of institutionalization, greater need for rehabilitation, and home care services, and higher costs . . . Thus, nurses are responsible for facilitating patients' recovery in less time for an increasingly older population at greater risk for functional decline" (Zalon, 2004, p. 99).
   b. Background of the problem: "Research has demonstrated that pain, depression, and fatigue occur after joint arthoroplasty and coronary artery bypass graft (CABG), and that they occur in relation to the functional status of older adults in residential care (Gallagher, Verma, &

Mossey, 2000; Liao & Ferrell, 2000; Redeker, 1993)" (Zalon, 2004, p. 99).
   c. Problem statement: "However, few studies have specifically examined pain, depression, and fatigue in relation to the recovery of older adults after their discharge to the community after major abdominal surgery. The extent of inadequate postoperative pain relief after discharge is not known" (Zalon, 2004, p. 99). This study includes 4 or 5 problem statements about what is not known on pp. 99 and 100. The one stated above is the most comprehensive.

2. Study purpose: "To determine whether pain, depression, and fatigue are significant factors in the return of older adults who had major abdominal surgery to functional status and self-perception of recovery in the first 3 months after discharge from the hospital" (Zalon, 2004, p. 99).

3. The problem and purpose are significant because of the increasing number of older adults in society and their expanding health needs, including the need for abdominal surgery. Care of the elderly requires a unique knowledge base for the nurse to facilitate their recovery and return to their homes in the most cost-effective way. Pain, fatigue, and depression are important variables to understand in promoting the elderly toward recovery and improved functional status.

4. Yes, the variables, population, and settings are identified.
   a. This is a predictive correlational study, and the dependent variables of pain, fatigue, and depression were used to predict two independent variables of functional status and perception of recovery.
   b. Populations: Older adults who had major abdominal surgery
   c. Settings: Hospital and patient homes after discharge

5. The problem and purpose are feasible because (1) the study was funded by the National Institute of Nursing Research (NINR) and an internal faculty research grant from the University of Scranton; (2) Zalon had previous research in this area and clinical expertise, as discussed in Chapter 2 of this study guide; (3) adequate subjects were available to participate in the study; (4) hospital personnel were supportive of the study; (5) no special equipment was needed for the study; and (5) the study was ethical and protected the rights of the subjects.

Going Beyond

Do the exercises as identified and seek feedback from peers and your instructor. Be sure to select a research problem and purpose that is of significance to nursing and of interest to you.

CHAPTER 6

Relevant Terms

Check the glossary in the back of your text for definitions.

Key Ideas

1. You could have chosen any five of the following:
   a. Clarify the research topic
   b. Clarify the research problem
   c. Verify the significance of the research problem
   d. Specify the purpose of the study
   e. Describe relevant studies
   f. Describe relevant theories
   g. Summarize current knowledge
   h. Facilitate development of the framework
   i. Specify research objectives, questions, or hypotheses
   j. Develop definitions of major variables
   k. Identify limitations and assumptions for the study
   l. Select a research design
   m. Identify methods of measurement
   n. Direct data collection and analysis
   o. Facilitate interpretation of findings
2. Advantages of electronic databases:
   a. Provide a large scope of available literature internationally
   b. Identify relevant sources quickly
   c. Print full-text versions of sources immediately
3. a. It helps you avoid going back along paths you have already searched.
   b. It helps you retrace your steps if need be.
   c. It helps you select new paths to search.
4. Theoretical; empirical
5. Primary
6. Computer; manual
7. a. Using the library
   b. Identifying relevant sources
   c. Locating research sources
   d. Summarizing the research literature
8. a. Catalog listings
   b. Indexes
   c. Abstracts
   d. Bibliographies
9. Cumulative Index to Nursing and Allied Health Literature (CINAHL)
10. a. Nursing and Allied Health (NAHL)
    b. MEDLINE (MEDical literature analysis and retrieval system onLINE)
11. *Annual Review of Nursing Research*
12. Synthesis
13. Store information related to literature sources and to provide in-text citations and reference lists in the correct format
14. a. Introduction
    b. Theoretical literature
    c. Empirical literature
    d. Summary
15. Key terms to direct the literature review include acute myocardial infarction symptoms, delay treatment for women, rate mortality and morbidity for women.
16. Key terms to direct the literature review include smoking revalence, Appalachian

states, heart disease rates, cancer rates, smoking cessation, transtheoretical model.

17. Key terms to direct the literature review include cancer-related pain, untreated pain, cancer pain management.

18. a. Limit to English language
    b. Limit the years of your search
    c. Limit the search to only papers that are research, are reviews, are published in consumer health journals, include abstracts, or are available in full text

19. You could identify any four of the following research journals:
    a. *Applied Nursing Research*
    b. *Image: Journal of Nursing Scholarship*
    c. *Nursing Research*
    d. *Research in Nursing & Health*
    e. *Scholarly Inquiry for Nursing Practice*
    f. *Western Journal of Nursing Research*

20. You could identify any three of the following journals:
    a. *Issues in Comprehensive Pediatric Nursing*
    b. *Journal of Transcultural Nursing*
    c. *Heart & Lung: Journal of Critical Care*
    d. *Journal of Nursing Education*
    e. *Birth*
    f. *Nursing Diagnosis*
    g. *Public Health Nursing*
    h. *The Diabetes Educator*
    i. *Maternal-Child Nursing Journal*
    j. *Journal of Nursing Education*

21. a. Introduction
    b. Methods
    c. Results
    d. Discussion

22. Skimming, comprehending, analyzing, and synthesizing

23. Paraphrase

Making Connections

Purpose of the Literature Review

1. e	3. f	5. b
2. d	4. a	6. c

Theoretical and Empirical Literature

1. T	5. T	9. T
2. E	6. E	10. T
3. E	7. E	11. E
4. T	8. E	

Primary and Secondary Sources

1. S	3. P	5. S
2. P	4. S	6. P

Exercises in Critique

1. a. Title of the journal
   b. Year the study was published
   c. Volume number of the journal
   d. Pages of the article
   e. Issue number of the journal
   f. Sethares and Elliott

2. Zalon, M.L. Correlates of recovery among older adults after major abdominal surgery. *Nursing Research, 53*(2), 99-106.

3. a. Title and pages of the article
   b. Volume number of the journal and pages of the article
   c. Year the article was published and volume and issue numbers of the journal

4. a. Literature Review
   b. Part of introduction
   c. No title, part of introduction

5. Yes. You might have identified any of the following: Baker, Andrew, Schrader, & Knight (2001); Barsevick, Pasacreta, & Orsi (1995); Chrsitensen & Kehlet (1993); DeCherney, Bachmann, Isaacson, & Gall (2002); Gallagher, Verma, & Mossey (2000); Mossey, Knott, & Craik (1990); Swan (1998); Zimmerman, Barnason, Brey, Catlin, & Nieveen (2002)

6. Yes, Levine (1991).

7. Secondary source

8. The reference dates range from 1971 to 2002. The article was published in 2004, so the author is citing current sources.

9. Sethares and Elliott clearly summarized the current knowledge base in intervention studies and transitional care models. These

are consistent with the problem and purpose of the study.

10. Yes. You might have listed: Rich, Beckham, Wittenberg, Leen, Freedland, & Carney (1995); Naylor & McCauley (1999); Bennett, Hays, Embree, Arnould (2000); Naylor, Brooten, Campbell, Jacobsen, Mezey, Pauly, et al (1999).
11. Becker (1974)
12. a. Primary source
    b. Secondary source
13. The reference dates range from 1974 to 2003. The 1974 publications are theoretical papers. Most of the studies cited are in the last 10 years. Thus the current literature is well covered in the literature review.
14. Yes, the knowledge base in pain, depression, and fatigue and their effects on recovery are carefully reviewed and examined, particularly for recovery for older adults.
15. Yes. You might have mentioned: Prochaska, DiClemente, & Norcross (1992); Murphy (1993); Davis (1997); Jackson (1995).
16. Yes. You might have mentioned: Watson (1988); Roy (1984); Neuman (1989); and Reed (1992).
17. a. Primary
    b. Secondary
18. The literature cited ranges from 1962 to 2001. Since the study was published in 2003, the studies cited are recent.
19. Yes. However, the knowledge base for African American women recovering from drug addiction was very limited. Knowledge of spirituality has been examined for a variety of situations, but none had examined spirituality in relation to recovery from drug addiction in women, particularly not African American women.

CHAPTER 7

Relevant Terms

Check the glossary in the back of your text for definitions.

Key Ideas

1. Organize what we know about a phenomenon
2. Determining the truth of each relational statement in the theory
3. Conceptual models
4. Theory
5. Effect size
6. Framework
7. Concepts
8. Constructs
9. Variable
10. Propositions
11. Hypotheses
12. Explain which concepts contribute to or partially cause an outcome
13. All of the major concepts in a theory or framework linked together by arrows expressing the proposed linkages between the concepts
14. Research tradition

Making Connections

1. c
2. b
3. e
4. f
5. a
6. i
7. h
8. d
9. g

Puzzles

Word Scramble

Many studies are required to validate all of the statements in a theory.

Secret Message

You need to determine links among the conceptual definitions, the variables in the study, and the related measurement methods.

Crossword Puzzle

Across
1. Conceptual model
4. Implicit
6. Framework
7 Hypothesis
11. Self-care
12. Abstract
13. Variable
14. Tradition

Down
1. Concrete
2. Theory testing
3. Map
5. Theory
8. Proposition
9. Statement
10. Adaptation

Exercises in Critique

1. Concepts:
   a. Recovery
   b. Energy
   c. Structural integrity
   d. Personal and social integrity
2. Conceptual definitions:
   a. Recovery—Improvement in functional status and the perception that one is recovering. In the context of Levine's (1991) Conservation Model, recovery is a return to wholeness that occurs by conservation of energy and restoration of integrity.
   b. Energy—Uses Levine's definition but does not provide it in the article.
   c. Structural integrity—Uses Levine's definition but does not provide it in the article.
   d. Personal and social integrity—Uses Levine's definition but does not provide it in the article.
3. Variables:
   a. Functional status
   b. Perception of recovery
   c. Pain
   d. Depression
   e. Fatigue
4. Relationship between concepts and variables:
   a. Energy
      • Pain
      • Depression
      • Fatigue
   b. Structural integrity
      • Pain
   c. Personal and social integrity
      • Depression
   d. Recovery
      • Functional status
      • Perception of recovery
5. Method used to measure each variable:
   a. Enforced Social Dependency Scale
   b. Self-Perception of Recovery
   c. Brief Pain Inventory
   d. Geriatric Depression Scale
   e. Modified Fatigue Symptom Checklist

6.

Concept	Variable(s)	Measurement Method(s)
Recovery	Functional status	Enforced Social Dependency Scale
	Perception of recovery	Self-Perception of Recovery After Surgery Rating Scale
Energy	Pain	Brief Pain Inventory
	Depression	Geriatric Depression Scale
	Fatigue	Modified Fatigue Symptom Checklist
Structural integrity	Pain	Brief Pain Inventory
Personal and social integrity	Depression	Geriatric Depression Scale

7. All of the study concepts are included in a statement. The measure of functional status is reflective of the concept of recovery. Energy, structural integrity and personal and social

integrity are measured in the negative, the extent to which they are not present, rather than the positive presence of the concept.

8. Statements:
   a. <u>Recovery</u> is a return to <u>wholeness</u> that occurs by <u>conservation of energy</u> and <u>restoration of integrity</u>.

      Conservation of Energy + Restoration of Integrity → Recovery → Wholeness

   b. When <u>pain</u> and <u>depressive symptoms</u> are decreased, <u>energy</u> is conserved.

      Pain ↓ + Depression ↓ → Energy ↑

   c. When <u>fatigue</u> is decreased, more <u>energy</u> is available to the individual.

      Fatigue ↓ → Energy ↑

   d. Acute <u>pain</u> depletes <u>energy</u> and generally indicates impaired <u>structural integrity</u> after surgery.

      Pain ↑ → Energy ↓ → Structural Integrity ↓

   e. Older patients are more likely to have persistent <u>pain</u>, to experience less relief from analgesics, and to use fewer analgesics.

      Age ↑ → Pain ↑

   f. None of the aforementioned studies examined the relation of <u>pain</u> to <u>functional status</u> in the first few months after discharge

      Pain ? → Functional Status?

   g. Retirement center residents whose <u>pain</u> interfered with their lives rated their health as worse, were more likely to be <u>depressed</u>, and had lower physical <u>functioning</u>.

      Pain ↑ → Depression ↑ + Functional Status ↓

   h. Older adults, because they are more likely to have unrelieved or persistent <u>pain</u> after surgery, are at greater risk for its interference with <u>function</u>, thus delaying <u>recovery</u>.

      Age ↑ → Functional Status ↓ → Recovery ↓

   i. <u>Depression</u> depletes the conservation of <u>personal integrity</u>.

      Depression ↑ → Personal Integrity ↓

   j. <u>Fatigue</u> is a manifestation of limited <u>energy</u> resources.

      Fatigue = Energy ↓

   k. It is not known to what extent postoperative <u>fatigue</u> is related to <u>functional status</u>.

      Fatigue ? ↔ Functional Status?

   l. Older adults may be more vulnerable to the effects of postoperative <u>fatigue</u> on <u>functional status</u>.

      Age ↑ + Fatigue ↑ → Functional Status ↓

When these relational statements are combined, they can be shown as a map expressing the existing knowledge base and providing some validity for the researcher's framework map shown below.

9. Links between propositions and hypotheses:
   a. Proposition: Pain ↑ → Depression ↑ + Functional Status ↓

   Age↑ + Fatigue ↑ → Functional Status ↓

   Research question: What is the relation of pain, depression, and fatigue to recovery?
10. The study used a correlational, predictive design to examine the relation of pain, depression, and fatigue to functional status and self-perception of recovery.
11. The researcher does not provide a conceptual map. A proposed map is provided below.

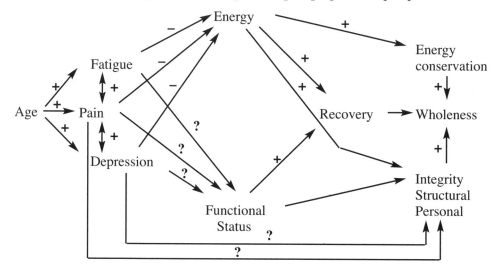

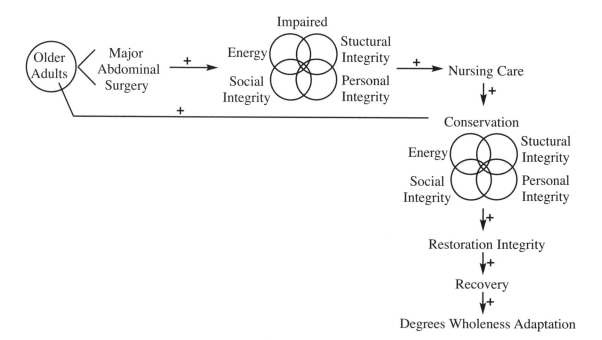

12. The author provides statements for each linkage on the map. References to support each linkage include:

    a. Recovery is a return to wholeness that occurs by conservation of energy and restoration of integrity (Levine, 1991).

    b. When pain and depressive symptoms are decreased, energy is conserved (Levine, 1991).

    c. When fatigue is decreased, more energy is available to the individual (Levine, 1991).

    d. Acute pain depletes energy and generally indicates impaired structural integrity after surgery. Cites sources indicating that unrelieved pain is a persistent problem during hospitalization for surgery and after discharge. Sources do not link pain to energy level or to impaired structural integrity (Devine et al., 1999; Moore, 1994; Redeker, 1993; Warfield & Kahn, 1995).

    e. Older patients are more likely to have persistent pain, to experience less relief from analgesics, and to use fewer analgesics (Lay, Puntillo, Miaskowski, & Wallhagen, 1996; MacIntyre & Jarvis, 1996).

    f. None of the aforementioned studies examined the relation of pain to functional status in the first few months after discharge.

    g. Retirement center residents whose pain interfered with their lives rated their health as worse, were more likely to be depressed and had lower physical functioning (Gallagher et al., 2000).

    h. Older adults, because they are more likely to have unrelieved or persistent pain after surgery, are at greater risk for its interference with function, thus delaying recovery.

    i. Depression depletes the conservation of personal integrity (Mulsant & Ganguli, 1999; Koenig, 1997; Pouger, Yersin, Wietlisbach, Bumand, & Bula, 2000).

    j. Fatigue is a manifestation of limited energy resources (Levine, 1991; Christensen & Kehlet, 1993; Rubin & Hotopf, 2002; Redeker, 1993; Zimmerman, Barnason, Bray, Catlin, & Nieveen, 2002; DeCherney, Bachmann, Isaacson, & Gall, 2002; Galloway, et al., 1997).

    k. It is not known to what extent postoperative fatigue is related to functional status (Westerblad and Allen, 2002; Liao and Ferrell, 2000).

    l. Older adults may be more vulnerable to the effects of postoperative fatigue on functional status (Westerblad and Allen, 2002; Liao and Ferrell, 2000).

13. The framework for Zalon's study is well stated. All of the expected components are present, other than a conceptual map. Linkages among the components of the framework are clearly delineated. Some of the linkages have not been validated in previous studies. Operationalization of some of the theoretical concepts is not strong, since it measures, in a sense, low levels of the concept rather than its fullness.

CHAPTER 8

Relevant Terms

General Concepts

1. b	3. a
2. d	4. c

Types of Hypotheses

1. h	4. e	7. d
2. g	5. c	8. f
3. b	6. a	

Types of Variables

1. a	3. f	5. e
2. d	4. c	6. b

Key Ideas

1. Objectives; questions; hypotheses
2. Independent; dependent
3. Directions
4. Null hypothesis
5. Contains variables that are measurable or manipulatable in the world
6. Treatment, intervention, experimental variable, or stimulus
7. Criterion, outcome variable, or response
8. Concepts
9. Confounding
10. Environmental
11. Sample characteristics

Making Connections

Types of Hypotheses

1. b, c, d, g
2. a, c, e, g
3. b, c, e, f
4. a, d, g, h
5. b, d, g, h
6. b, c, d, g
7. a, c, e, g
8. b, c, e, f
9. a, c, e, g
10. b, d, g, h
11. Increased age, decreased family support, and decreased health status are related to decreased self-care abilities of nursing home residents.
12. Low-back massage is no more effective in decreasing perceptions of low-back pain than no massage in patients with chronic low-back pain.

Types of Variables

1. a
2. b
3. c
4. a
5. a or b
6. b
7. c

8. c
9. a
10. b
11. a
12. a

Exercises in Critique

Sethares and Elliott Study

1. Sethares and Elliott (2004) included three research questions and three hypotheses. "The following research questions are the basis for the study: 1. Do individuals who receive the tailored message intervention have lower HF readmission rates than a control group at 3 months? 2. Do individuals who receive a tailored message intervention report better quality of life at baseline and 1 month after discharge than a control group? 3. What is the effect of the tailored message intervention on the perceived benefit and barrier beliefs of the treatment group at baseline, 1 week, and 1 month? There were three hypotheses for the study. The first two hypotheses were that persons who received the intervention would have lower HF readmission rates and report better quality of life. The third hypothesis was that intervention subjects would report fewer barriers and more benefits to performing self-care of HF after receiving the tailored message intervention (Sethares & Elliott, 2004, p. 251).

2. The study really does not need both questions and hypotheses; these are redundant. Since this is a quasi-experimental study, the hypotheses are most appropriate to guide the study. Three separately stated hypotheses would be the clearest. The hypotheses provided are reflective of the study purpose, clearly indicate the focus of the study, include the study variables, and identify the proposed outcomes for the study.

3. Sethares and Elliott (2004) have one independent variable of tailored message and four dependent variables of readmission

rate for HF, reported quality of life, perceived barrier beliefs, and perceived benefit beliefs.

4. Independent variable: Tailored message intervention
   a. Conceptual definition: Tailored message is an intervention "focused on decreasing client-identified barriers to self-care. Individualized teaching by a nurse focused on enhancing the benefits and decreasing the barriers to self-care of a person with HF . . . By changing perceived beliefs [benefits and barriers] related to self-care, it is anticipated that persons with HF will improve self-care behaviors, which may lead to improved quality of life and lower readmission rates" (Sethares & Elliott, 2004, p. 251).
   b. Operational definition: The tailored message was "based on the perceived benefits and barriers to self-care of HF that were identified by persons with HF" (Sethares & Elliott, 2004, p. 254). The specifics of the intervention are provided under the heading Intervention (pp. 254-255), and the tailored messages for diet and medications are in Table III (p. 255) in the article.

5. The demographic variables are identified in Tables I and II and include the following: age, NYHA, EF, number of comorbidities, education, marital status, race, gender, medications, and VNA services.

Wright Study

1. Wright (2003) used the purpose to guide her study and had no objectives, questions, or hypotheses.
2. The purpose of this study is clearly stated and provides direction to the study. Often in qualitative studies, the research purpose is used to direct the study. Qualitative studies sometimes have research questions and occasionally objectives but do not include hypotheses.

3. Wright (2004) has one research concept: lived experience of spirituality in recovery from substance abuse.

4. Lived experience of spirituality in recovery from substance abuse
   a. Conceptual definition: This definition was provided in the results section of the article in Tables 1 and 2 (Wright, 2003, pp. 177-178), which include the major meaning units and themes in the study. Often in qualitative research, the theoretical understanding of the concept is provided in the results and discussion section of the article.
   b. Operational definition: The lived experience of spirituality is measured by in-depth, unstructured interviews with subjects recovering from substance abuse.

5. Demographic variables included in this study were age, marital status, religious affiliation, age of onset of substance abuse, past legal problems, and abstinence time in years or months (Wright, 2003, p. 176).

Zalon Study

1. Zalon (2004, p. 100) stated: "Therefore, the following research question was addressed: What is the relation of pain, depression, and fatigue to recovery, as measured by functional status and self-perception of recovery in older adults who have had major abdominal surgery?"
2. The research question is really just a restatement of the study purpose and does not add clarity to the focus of the study. The study has a predictive correlational design, and it might have been best to state hypotheses that could be tested in the study. The hypotheses might have been stated as: (a) Pain, depression, and fatigue are predictive of functional status in elderly adults following abdominal surgery and (b) Pain, depression, and fatigue are predictive of self-perception of recovery in elderly adults following abdominal surgery.

3. Dependent variables of pain, depression, and fatigue were used to predict the two independent variables of functional status and self-perception of recovery.
4. Depression
   a. Conceptual definition: "Depression depletes the conservation of personal integrity, which results in impaired wholeness and increased time to recovery" (Zalon, 2004, p. 100).
   b. Operational definition: "Depression was measured with the short form of the Geriatric Depression Scale" (Zalon, 2004, p. 101).
5. Demographic and Medical Record Data section in the article clearly lists the demographic variables: "Background data included age, gender, education, marital status, religion, race, ethonocultural identification . . . length of stay, diagnostic related group, discharge medication, and activity restrictions" (Zalon, 2004, p. 101).

Going Beyond

Develop objectives, questions, or hypotheses for a proposed study and conceptually and operationally define the variables. Share these with peers and your instructor for feedback.

CHAPTER 9

Relevant Terms

1. o	10. j	19. z
2. a	11. e	20. y
3. p	12. s	21. n
4. r	13. t	22. l
5. f	14. w	23. x
6. q	15. h	24. i
7. g	16. c	25. d
8. k	17. u	26. m
9. b	18. v	

Key Ideas

1. a. Principle of respect for persons
   b. Principle of beneficence
   c. Principle of justice
2. Children (minors), mentally impaired individuals (mentally ill and those with dementia), unconscious patients, terminally ill patients, and those confined to institutions (prisoners)
3. Competent
4. Assent
5. a. Best interest standard: The decision to participate in the study is based on what is therapeutically in the best interest of the mentally incompetent patient and also to ask the patient for his or her assent to participate in the study.
   b. Substituted judgment standard: The decision to participate in the study is based on what the patient would have probably wanted if he or she were mentally competent to give consent and also to ask the patient to assent to participate in the study.
6. Qualitative
7. a. Disclosure of essential study information to the subject
   b. Comprehension of this information by the subject
   c. Competency of the subject to give consent
   d. Voluntary consent by the subject to participate in the study
8. You could have identified any of the following:
   a. Introduction of the research activities
   b. Statement of the research purpose
   c. Explanation of study procedures
   d. Description of risks and discomforts
   e. Description of benefits
   f. Disclosure of alternatives
   g. Assurance of anonymity and confidentiality
   h. Offer to answer questions
   i. Option to withdraw

9. Voluntary
10. Institutional review board
11. Short written consent form, long written consent form, tape recording of consent process, or a videotape of the consent process
12. Research (or scientific) misconduct
13. Promoting the integrity of biomedical and behavior research in approximately 4000 institutions worldwide
14. You could have identified any of the following:
    a. Defining research misconduct
    b. Developing policies aimed at preventing misconduct and promoting the conduct of ethical research
    c. Identifying mechanisms to distribute the policy to scientists
    d. Designating membership of committees investigating research misconduct
    e. Identifying the administrative actions for acts of research misconduct
    f. Developing a process for notifying funding agencies and journals
    g. Providing for public disclosure of the incidents of scientific misconduct
    h. Identifying legal ramifications
    i. Prevention and the role of peer review
15. a. Exempt from review
    b. Expedited review
    c. Complete or full review
16. a. Should animals be used as subjects in a research project?
    b. If animals are used in research, what mechanisms ensure that they are treated humanely?
17. American Association for Accreditation of Laboratory Animal Care (AAALAC)
18. To determine the benefit-risk ratio, you need to assess the benefits and risks of the sampling method, consent process, procedures, and outcomes of the study. Informed consent must be obtained from the subjects, and selection and treatment of the subjects during the study must be fair. The type of knowledge generated from the study also needs to be examined to determine how this knowledge will influence nursing practice.
19. You need the approval of the school to conduct the study. You need to obtain an informed consent from the children's parents or legal guardians and assent of each child.
20. Protected health information

Making Connections

Levels of Discomfort or Harm

1. b	5. e	8. d
2. a	6. b or c	9. e
3. c	7. a	10. c
4. c or d		

Unethical Studies

1. b	5. c	8. b
2. c	6. a	9. a
3. d	7. d	10. c
4. b		

Puzzles

Crossword Puzzle

Across
1. Confidentiality
4. Institutional review
6. Autonomous
7. Nuremberg
10. Self-determination
11. Ethics
13. Assent
14. Privacy
15. Anonymous

Down
2. Fair treatment
3. Risk
5. IRB
8. Deception
9. Consent
12. Children

Exercises in Critique

1. Sethares and Elliott (2004) received approval from the institutional review board (IRB) at the community hospital where the study was conducted. "After stabilization of HF [heart failure], hospitalized subjects were invited to participate in the study, and written informed consent was obtained" (p. 254). The study was ethical because the researchers obtained institutional approval

from the hospital and written informed consent from the subjects who voluntarily participated in the study. In additional, the potential subjects were not approached until their HF was stabilized, which strengthens the ethics of this study. The results and discussion sections of the study protect the privacy of the subjects and do not reflect the protected health information of any one subject.

2. Wright (2003) indicated that the purpose of the study was explained and informed consent was obtained from the subjects. The subjects were also given a rationale for the researcher's interest in the phenomenon studied. Wright recognized that "the recall of painful memories can trigger anxiety and other emotional distress. Therefore, the emotional state of each participant was evaluated throughout the interviews by stopping when the participant was upset and offering support" (p. 177). Thus Wright (2003) documented the informed consent process and the method for protecting subjects from discomfort and harm. However, she did not document the institutional review of this study by the shelter where the data were collected or by the National Institute of Health (NIH) that provided support for the study (or at least was the site of the study). The ethics of this study would be strengthened by the inclusion of the IRB process that was implemented before the study was conducted.

3. Zalon (2004) clearly identifies the IRB approval, informed consent process, and the protection of potential subjects from discomfort and harm for her study. "Institutional review board approval was obtained at each site . . . Consents were obtained postoperatively, allowing for the inclusion of participants who had undergone emergency surgery . . . Nurses were interviewed to determine whether the patients were medically unstable or whether they had experienced episodes of delirium in the pre-

ceding 24 hours. Patients were approached about participation while resting comfortably" (pp. 101-102). The results and discussion sections of the research report protect the privacy of the subjects, and their protected health information is not revealed.

Going Beyond

Use the content in Chapter 9 to discuss the benefit-risk ratio for a proposed study, develop a consent form, and complete an IRB form.

CHAPTER 10

Relevant Terms

Check the glossary in the back of your text for definitions.

Key Ideas

1. Effects
2. Cause; effect; cause
3. Biases
4. Control
5. Treatment
6. Threats to validity
7. Cause and effect
8. Comparisons
9. Comparisons

Making Connections

Research Design Terms

1. d	4. g	7. a
2. h	5. i	8. b
3. f	6. e	9. c

Design Control Methods

1. h	5. j	8. m
2. b	6. d	9. e
3. f	7. a	10. l
4. k		

Puzzles

Word Scramble

Just as the blueprint for a house must be individualized to the specific house being built, so must the design be made specific to a study.

Secret Message

The purpose of a design is to set up a situation that maximizes the possibilities of obtaining accurate answers to objectives, questions, or hypotheses.

Crossword Puzzle

Across	Down
1. Matching	2. Heterogeneity
4. Comparisons	3. Map
7. Effect	5. Manipulation
8. Counterbalancing	6. Sample
10. Equivalence	8. Control
12. Treatment	9. Blocking
16. Validity	11. Correlational
17. Threat	13. Random
18. Probability	14. Bias
19. Design	15. Descriptive
20. Stratification	17. Trend
21. Experimental	

Exercises in Critique

1. Sources of bias:
   a. Zalon's study
      - Sample not randomly selected: subjects volunteering may have been different from those who did not volunteer.
      - 28.5% of patients approached declined to participate in the study. Those patients who refused may have been different from those who agreed to participate, resulting in a bias in the sampling.
      - The sample was almost totally non-Hispanic White and thus not representative of minority populations.
      - Since only patients who were discharged directly home were included in the study, there is a bias toward patients who were recovering well enough to go directly home.
   b. Sethares and Elliott's study
      - Sample not randomly selected: subjects volunteering may have been different from those who did not volunteer.
      - Subjects were limited to patients who planned to be discharged home, rather than a nursing home or other facility. This strategy provided a more homogeneous sample but suggests a possible bias of the patients having a stronger support system than those who were not discharged home. A strong support system might have altered the perception of benefits and barriers.
      - The subjects were obtained from a single hospital.
2. Methods of control:
   a. Zalon's study
      - Controlling environment: All subjects were approached about participation in the study after surgery when they were in a comfortable situation.
      - Controlling extraneous variables: Subjects were required to be alert and oriented, able to speak and read English, and be accessible by phone.
      - Homogeneity: Subjects were limited to patients 60 years of age or older who had abdominal surgery.
      - Controlling measurement: Instruments with documented validity and reliability and use with older subjects were used for measurement.
   b. Sethares and Elliott's study
      - Controlling measurement: Valid and reliable instruments were used.

- Controlling extraneous variables: Subjects were randomly assigned to treatment and control groups.
- Homogeneity: Subjects had documented diagnoses of systolic or diastolic heart failure confirmed by echocardiography and were free from serious cognitive deficits.

3. Populations generalized to:
   a. Zalon's study—White patients 60 years of age or older, with at least a high school education, who have had abdominal surgery.
   b. Sethares and Elliott's study—Adults with a primary diagnosis of chronic heart failure who were discharged home. No information is provided on subject's ethnicity or socioeconomic status.
4. Threats to external validity:
   a. Zalon's study—Generalization limited to White, English-speaking people over the age of 60 with at least a high school education who have telephones and receive hospital care at a community hospital.
   b. Sethares and Elliott's study—Generalization limited to English-speaking adults with heart failure who are free from serious cognitive deficits and anticipate returning to a community setting. There were only six African Americans included in the study and no mention of Hispanic subjects. Therefore generalization to minority groups would be questionable. Lack of information on socioeconomic status makes generalizability to low-income patients questionable.

CHAPTER 11

Relevant Terms

Check the glossary in the back of your text for definitions.

Key Ideas

1. To achieve greater control and thus improve the validity of the study in examining the research problem
2. Nursing philosophy
3. Time
4. Self-report
5. The full range of scores possible on the variables being measured
6. Causality
7. Highly, not highly
8. Improved outcomes of the experimental group
9. The actual effects of the experimental treatment can be detected by measurement of the dependent variable
10. Random selection
11. Nested variables
12. Valid answers to the questions that have been posed

Making Connections

Designs

1. g
2. h
3. b, c

4. a
5. i

6. j
7. f

Mapping the Design

1. Treolar (1994):

	Pretest) (before heelstick)	**During heelstick**	**Treatment (Pacifier inserted)**	**Posttest (5 min after heelstck)**
Experimental Group NNS Infants	O_1	O_2	T	O_3
Control Group ONNS Infants	O_1	O_2		O_3

Note: O = Trancutaneous oxygen and behavioral state data

2. Guiffre, Heidenreich, and Pruitt (1994):

	Pretest Temperature Measured	**Treatment**	**Repeated Posttests Temperature Measured**
Radiant heat group	O_1	T_1	$O_2\ O_3\ O_4\ O_5\ O_6\ O_7$
Forced warm air group	O_1	T_2	$O_2\ O_3\ O_4\ O_5\ O_6\ O_7$
Warm blanket group	O_1	T_3	$O_2\ O_3\ O_4\ O_5\ O_6\ O_7$

Exercises in Critique

1. Design:
   a. Zalon's study—predictive correlational
   b. Sethares and Elliott's study—randomized control trial
2. Comparisons:
   a. Zalon's study
      - Pain at 3-5 days and 1 month
      - Pain at 1 month and 3 months
      - Pain at 3-5 days and 3 months
      - Depression at 3-5 days and 1 month
      - Depression at 1 month and 3 months
      - Depression at 3-5 days and 3 months
      - Fatigue at 3-5 days and 1 month
      - Fatigue at 1 month and 3 months
      - Fatigue at 3-5 days and 3 months
      - Functional status at 3-5 days and 1 month
      - Functional status at 1 month and 3 months
      - Functional status at 3-5 days and 3 months
   b. Sethares and Elliott's study
      - Health Belief Scale Scores of experimental group during hospitalization and 7-10 days later
      - Quality of Life Scores 1 month after hospitalization comparing experimental group and control group
      - Readmission rate at 3 months comparing experimental and control groups
      - Readmission rate with quality of life
      - Readmission rate with health beliefs 7-10 days after discharge in experimental group

3. Strengths of the design:
   a. Zalone's study
      - Data collection across 4 time periods
      - Subjects obtained from 3 community hospitals
      - Screening for cognitive status before selecting as subjects
      - Training of data collectors
      - Use of same data collector for a subject across time
      - Sample size of 192
      - Comparison of individuals who declined to participate with participants.
   b. Sethares and Elliott's study
      - Carefully designed intervention
      - Description of care received by control subjects
      - Protocol reviewed with research nurses weekly to maintain consistency in treatment
      - Random assignment to groups
      - Interview and measurements guided by theoretical framework

CHAPTER 12

Relevant Terms

Check the glossary in the back of your text for definitions.

Key Ideas

1. The end results of patient care
2. a. The Hospital and Medical Facilities Study Section
   b. The Nursing Study Section
3. Medical Outcomes Study (MOS)
4. a. The effect of nursing interventions on medical outcomes
   b. The effect of staffing patterns on medical outcomes
   c. The effects of nursing practice delivery models on medical outcomes

5. a. Coordination of care
   b. Counseling
   c. Referrals
6. a. Do patients benefit from the care provided?
   b. What treatments work best?
   c. Has the patient's functional status improved? According to whose viewpoint?
   d. Are health care resources well spent?
7. Incorporate available evidence on health outcomes into sets of recommendations concerning appropriate management strategies for patients with the studied conditions
8. Inclusion of nursing data in the large databases used to analyze outcomes
9. Clearly linked; process; caused
10. Subjects of care
11. a. Clinical guidelines
    b. Critical paths
    c. Care maps
12. Large heterogeneous
13. a. Information about the patient such as disease severity, comorbidity, and types of outcomes
    b. Processes of care provided
    c. Patient status over time
    d. Follow-up information
14. a. Decisions can be quantified.
    b. All possible courses of action can be identified and evaluated.
    c. The different values of outcomes, viewed from the perspective of the physician, patient, payer, and administrator can be examined.
    d. The analysis allows selection of an optimal course of therapy.
15. a. What proportion of people experiencing a specific cluster of symptoms were diagnosed (correctly or not) as having a particular condition, and of this group, who received what treatment?
    b. Should a treatment or procedure have been performed?

c. Did persons with a particular diagnosis receive appropriate treatment?

d. What proportion of people with the cluster of symptoms received no treatment?

16. a. There is no clearly superior treatment for all individuals with a given problem.

b. There are a number of treatments with some proved efficacy that are relatively comparable in their effectiveness for undifferentiated groups of subjects.

c. There is evidence of differential outcome either within or across treatments for defined subtypes of clients.

17. Most consistent with nursing theory and practice

18. Change across time in subjects

19. American Nurses Association

20. a. In change, regression toward the mean is an unavoidable law of nature.

b. The difference score between pre- and postmeasurement is unreliable.

c. ANCOVA is the way to analyze change.

d. Two points (pre- and posttest) are adequate for the study of change.

e. The correlation between change and initial level is always negative.

21. a. Mean improvement score for all patients' treatment

b. The percentage of patients that improve

c. Whether all patients improve slightly, or there is a divergence among patients, with some improving greatly while others do not improve at all

d. Characteristics of patients who experience varying degrees of improvement

e. Characteristics of outliers

22. a. Variance

b. Comorbidities

c. Identify at-risk patients

Making Connections

1. h   6. l   10. a
2. e   7. m   11. d
3. j   8. i   12. g
4. c   9. f   13. k
5. b

Puzzles

Word Scramble

The momentum propelling outcomes research is coming from policy makers, insurers, and the public.

Secret Message

The strategies used in outcome research are, to some extent, a departure from the accepted scientific method.

Crossword Puzzle

Across
1. Standard of care
4. Cost benefit
6. Patient
8. Person
11. Cohort
16. Numerical method
20. Efficiency
21. Variance
22. Individual
23. Research tradition

Down
2. Out of pocket cost
3. Measurement error
5. Structures of care
7. Geographic
9. Intermediate end point
10. Providers of care
12. Opportunity cost
13. Sampling error
14. Subjects of care
15. Primordial cell
17. Multilevel
18. Aggregate
19. Small area

CHAPTER 13

Relevant Terms

Check the glossary in the back of your text for definitions.

Key Ideas

1. Designing and testing nursing interventions
2. True experiment
3. a. Single act
   b. Series of actions at a given point in time
   c. Series of actions over time
   d. Series of acts performed collaboratively with other professionals
4. clinical trial
5. explain why the intervention causes changes in outcomes, how it does so, or both
6. all groups that will be affected by the change
7. a. the components, intensity, and duration required
   b. the human and material resources needed
   c. the procedures to be followed to produce the desired outcomes
8. amount, frequency, and duration
9. independent
10. confounding variables

Making Connections

Designing an Intervention

1. e	5. c	8. f
2. b	6. i	9. j
3. a	7. h	10. g
4. d		

Puzzles

Word Scramble

Interventions must be described more broadly as all of the actions required to address a particular problem.

Secret Message

There is currently little consistency in the performance of an intervention.

Crossword Puzzle

Across	Down
1. Treatment matching	2. Adaptation
3. Moderator variable	4. Key informat
6. Intensity	5. Prescriptive theory
8. Disadvantaged group	7. Stakeholder
12. Intervener	9. Extraneous factors
13. Complexity	10. Logical positivist
15. Effectiveness	11. Taxonomy
16. Dose	12. Intervention
17. Strength	14. True experiment
18. Integrity	
19. Reinvention	
20. Duration	
21. Observation system	
22. Intermediate outcome	

Exercises in Critique

Note: Although this study was not designed using an intervention theory approach, the authors do describe the intervention in their study sufficiently to allow you to critique the intervention.

1. No, the intervention is not sufficiently described to allow implementation of the intervention.
2. The intervention is theory-based but not in the manner of intervention theory methods.

CHAPTER 14

Relevant Terms

1. j	6. f	11. d
2. a	7. m	12. e
3. n	8. i	13. h
4. g	9. l	14. c
5. k	10. b	15. o

Key Ideas

1. Elements; subjects
2. Target population
3. Sample; accessible population; target population
4. a. Compare the demographic characteristics of the sample to those of the target population or the samples of similar previous studies.
   b. Compare mean sample values of study variables to the values of the target population determined from previous research.
   c. Determine sample mortality
   d. Evaluate the possibilities of systematic bias in the sample in terms of the setting, characteristics of the sample, and ranges of values on measured variables.
5. The expected difference in values that occurs when different subjects from the same sample are examined
6. Sampling frame
7. Strategies used to obtain a sample for a study
8. You could choose any of the following:
   a. Did the researcher successfully implement the sampling plan?
   b. Was the sampling plan effective in achieving representativeness of the target population?
   c. Were the subjects selected from a sampling frame?
   d. What sampling method was used to determine the sample?
   e. Were the subjects randomly selected?
   f. Was power analysis used to determine sample size?
   g. What sample size was achieved?
   h. Were the characteristics of the sample consistent with the characteristics of the accessible and the target populations?
9. Homogeneous
10. Heterogeneous
11. Sample criteria
12. Sample characteristics
13. Sample mortality
14. Random
15. Nonrandom
16. a. Simple random sampling
    b. Stratified random sampling
    c. Cluster sampling
    d. Systematic sampling
17. Probability
18. a. Convenience sampling
    b. Quota sampling
    c. Purposive sampling
    d. Network sampling
19. Nonprobability
20. Accidental sampling
21. Judgmental sampling
22. Power analysis
23. Differences or relationships
24. 0.8
25. Power analysis
26. Null hypothesis
27. a. Effect size of a study
    b. Type of study
    c. Number of variables
    d. Measurement sensitivity
    e. Data analysis techniques
28. a. Purpose sampling
    b. Network sampling
    c. Theoretical sampling
29. Purpose
30. a. Scope of the study
    b. Nature of the topic studied
    c. Quality of the data collected
    d. Study design
31. a. Natural settings
    b. Partially controlled settings
    c. Highly controlled settings
32. Natural
33. Highly controlled
34. Partially controlled
35. Inclusion; exclusion

Making Connections

Sampling Methods

1. f	6. g	11. f
2. b	7. h	12. c
3. c	8. b	13. d
4. a	9. e	14. i
5. i	10. d	15. f

Types of Settings

1. a	4. c
2. b	5. a
3. b or c	

Puzzles

Crossword Puzzle

Across
2. Comparison group
5. Random
6. Power analysis
7. Elements
9. Sampling methods
11. Bias
12. Accessible
13. Target
14. Network
15. Purposive

Down
1. Criteria
3. Probability
4. Sample size
5. Representative
8. Subjects
10. Population

Exercises in Critique

Sethares and Elliott (2004) Study

1. Population: Adults with a primary diagnosis of chronic heart failure

2. Sample inclusion criteria were as follows: "(1) primary diagnosis of either systolic or diastolic HF listed in the medical record, confirmed by the presence of symptoms of HF for 3 months or longer; (2) echocardiography for confirmation of ejection fraction; (3) English speaking; (4) freedom from serious cognitive deficits, as determined by the Mini Mental Status Exam; and (5) anticipated return to a community setting, rather than long-term care" (Sethares & Elliott, 2004, p. 252).

3. Sample or demographic characteristics are presented in Table I (p. 252) and Table II (p. 253) in the article.

4. Sample size was 70. ". . a power analysis with an effect size of .35, an alpha of .05, and a power of .80" was conducted (Sethares & Elliott, 2004, p. 252).

5. The sample size was adequate to examine most of the variables in this quasi-experimental study, since most of the findings were significant. Power analysis indicated that the sample size was adequate to detect differences if they existed. In the power table on p. 721 of your text, an effect size of 0.34, alpha = 0.05, and a sample of 70 yields a power of 0.90, which is more than adequate to detect the significant differences in the sample. Sethares and Elliott (2004, p. 252) stated that "the sample size provided adequate power for all outcome variables."

6. Sample mortality was 18 subjects (8 subjects withdrew and 10 subjects died), or 25.7%. "A t test was run to compare the 2 groups of patients (those who died within 3 months of the discharge and those who survived) . . . There were no significant differences on any of the measures between the 2 groups" (Sethares & Elliott, 2004, p. 252). This indicates the researchers did attempt to determine whether the mortality rate had an impact on the two groups (treatment and control) and none was found. This strengthens the sampling plan and indicates less potential for sampling error.

7. Nonprobability convenience sampling was used in this study.

8. Because the sample is not random, this has a potential to decrease its representativeness of the target population. However, actively recruiting subjects and including all subjects that met the sample criteria increases the representativeness of this sample. The sample size of 70 is a strength, but the 25.7% mortality rate decreases the representativeness of the sample. The sample was

obtained from one community hospital in the Northeast, and this decreases the representativeness of the sample also.

9. Because the sample is nonrandom, the mortality is high, and the study involved only one setting, the findings could be generalized to the accessible population but probably not the target population. However, the fact that these findings are consistent with an extensive number of other studies in this area increases the generalizability of the findings.

Wright (2003) Study

1. Population was African American women recovering from substance abuse.

2. Sample criteria: "Each participant met the following criteria: over 18 years of age; identified herself as an African American woman; substance free status for at least 1 year; able to participate and engage in interviews of 1 to 2 hours in length; expressed interest in participating in the study; not currently being treated for psychotic disorders; and was able to read and write in the English language. There was no length of substance abuse to enter the study" (Wright, 2003, p. 176).

3. Sample characteristics: "There were 15 participants who ranged from 29 to 49 years of age. With respect to marital status, the majority—eight of the participants—were never married, whereas six were divorced and one currently married . . . All the participants reported an increase in their spirituality since becoming drug free. All participants identified their higher power as God or Jesus Christ.

   Of the participants 12 began using substances between the ages of 5 to 12, with all having some form of structured treatment for substance abuse. A majority of the participants reported having past legal problems. With respect to abstinence eight participants reported 7-12 years of drug free

status and seven having 15-39 months of substance free status" (Wright, 2003, p. 176).

4. Sample size was 15 participants. No power analysis was used since this is a qualitative study and sample size is determined by factors other than a power analysis (Burns & Grove, 2005).

5. The sample size does seem adequate for this phenomenological study since data saturation was reached with no new themes appearing and various perspectives of the phenomenon of recovery from substance abuse were obtained. Wright (2003, p. 176) stated that "The number of participants was determined by the number of persons required to permit an in-depth exploration and obtain a clear understanding of the phenomenon of interest from various perspectives. This occurred with 15 participants when data saturation was achieved, with no new themes or essences emerging from the participants and the data were repeating."

6. No sample mortality is mentioned.

7. Nonprobability network sampling method was used. "Participants were recruited from a women's shelter with the help of a colleague as contact person, from church support groups within the community by the researcher who made church members aware of the study and the search for participants, and through networking, whereby each participant interviewed suggested the name of a potential new participant" (Wright, 2003, p. 176).

8. Representativeness of the sample is not a major focus of qualitative research. The focus is on understanding the specific study subjects and less on their representativeness of a target population. Wright did indicate "the study limitations, however, were the researcher having worked in psychiatry and substance abuse for many years observed a difference in the lives of African American women who had incorporated a spiritual belief in their recover process. Most of the participants were recruited from faith-based

women's shelter and church support groups; therefore, it was known that their belief was in God" (Wright, 2003. p. 183). This indicates the subjects in the sample were those with a faith base and are not representative of those women recovering from substance abuse who do not have a faith base.

9. Generalization of findings is not the focus of qualitative research. The focus is on understanding the phenomenon of recovery from substance abuse by African American women in a selected sample.

Zalon (2004) Study

1. Population was older adults experiencing major abdominal surgery

2. Inclusion sample criteria: "The criteria for inclusion in the study required the subject to be alert and oriented, able to speak and read English, and accessible by telephone" (Zalon, 2004, p. 101). Exclusion sample criteria: "Those who had laparoscopic surgery, neurologic dysfunction, a psychotic disorder, or surgery specifically for cancer were excluded" (Zalon, 2004, p. 101).

3. The study had a section entitled Demographic and Medical Record Data with the following demographic variables identified: "Background data included age, gender, education, marital status, religion, race, ethnocultural identification, previous pain, previous pain medication experience, depression treatment, occupation, living arrangements, and household income . . . height, weight, length of stay, diagnostic related group, discharge medication, and activity restrictions" (Zalon, 2004, p. 101). The sample characteristics were presented on p. 102 of the article: "The age of participants ranged from 60 to 87 . . . Those living alone comprised 29.5% of the sample."

4. Sample size was 192 male and female patients 60 years of age or older. No power analysis was mentioned to determine sample size.

5. The sample size appeared to be adequate due to the significance of the findings in the study. All variables were significantly related as predicted by the study framework and used to form two strong predictive formulas.

6. The sample mortality was 31 subjects (16%) at the start of the study. "Two persons withdrew consent during the initial interview; 13 subsequently had a change in discharge plans from home to another type of healthcare facility; 10 did not want to be bothered after discharge; 4 stated that they were "too sick"; 1 could not be reached; and 1 died" (Zalon, 2004, p. 102). As the study progressed over the 3 months, a total of 66 subjects (34%) did not continue the study. Thus the study had a high mortality rate.

7. Nonprobability sampling and the sampling method is sample of convenience.

8. The representativeness of the sample is limited by the large number of individuals who refused to participate in the study, and those who refused participation were significantly different from those who did participate. Zalon (2004, p. 102) indicated that a total of "295 persons met the criteria. Of these, 192 consented, 84 refused, and 19 were missed. Those who refused to participate were significantly older than those who consented (mean, 75 vs. 71.2 years; t = 4.28). The most common reasons for refusal were related to the person's perception of well-being (too sick, too depressed, not up to it, too weak) (n = 15) followed by a desire not to be bothered (n = 6)." The high sample mortality (34%) also decreased the sample's representativeness of the target population. The final sample was 129, which is a substantial sample size, which increases it representativeness.

9. The generalization of the study findings is decreased by the nonprobabilty sampling method, high sample mortality, and the high refusal rate of the subjects discussed previously. However, because these study findings were consistent with the findings of other studies, this increases the generalizability of the findings. The findings can be generalized to the accessible population but probably not to the target population, and additional research is needed in this problem area.

Study Settings

1. b, a   Sethares and Elliott (2004) used a partially controlled setting of a single community hospital where the environment was controlled for the implementation of the treatment and a natural setting of the subjects' homes following discharge.
2. a   Wright (2003) used natural settings of a women's shelter and church community support groups.
3. b, a   Zalon (2004) conducted her study over 3 months and used both hospital and patient home settings.

CHAPTER 15

Relevant Terms

Check the glossary in the back of your text for definitions.

Key Ideas

1. Trustworthy
2. True
3. Error
4. Direct
5. Indirect
6. 0.80
7. a.   Variations in administration of the measurement procedure
   b.   Subjects completing a paper-and-pencil scale accidentally marking the wrong column

c.   Punching the wrong key while entering data into the computer
8. a.   A weight scale that reads higher than it should
   b.   A thermometer that is not calibrated
   c.   Failure to count two exam questions in calculating exam grades

Making Connections

Error Types

1. b
2. b
3. a
4. b
5. a

Measurement Levels

1. c
2. a
3. b
4. c
5. a
6. b
7. c

Reliability or Validity Types

1. f
2. m
3. h
4. b
5. e
6. k
7. a
8. g
9. i
10. j
11. c
12. l
13. d

Puzzles

Word Scramble

There is no perfect measure.

Secret Message

Reliability testing needs to be performed on each instrument used in a study.

Crossword Puzzle

Across	**Down**
1. Collect	2. Equivalence
3. Mail	4. Instrument
6. Measurement	5. Data
10. Rating	7. Reliability
12. Stability	8. True score
13. Rare	9. Age
14. Ratio	11. Precision

Across	Down
16. Scales	12. Score
17. Error	15. Observe
18. Idea	20. Precision
19. Open	23. Interval
21. Place	25. Stress
22. Interview	26. Setting
24. Accuracy	27. Talk
25. Sensitivity	
28. Questionnaire	
29. Likert	
30. Ordinal	
31. Ask	
32. Nominal	

Exercises in Critique

1. Measurement of variables:

Zalon's study

Variable	Method of Measurement	Directness
Pain	Brief Pain Inventory	I
Depression	Geriatric Depression Scale	I
Fatigue	Modified Fatigue Symptom Checklist	I
Functional status	Enforced Social Dependency Scale	I
Self-perception of recovery after surgery	Rating scale	I

Sethares and Elliott's study

Variable	Method of Measurement	Directness
Heart failure readmission rates	Counting total number of admissions for HF in each group during the 3-month study interval	D
Quality of life	Minnesota Living with Heart Failure questionnaire	I
Benefits and barriers	Health Beliefs Scales	I

2. Reliability and validity of measures:

Zalon's study

a. Measure—Brief Pain Inventory

Type of Reliability or Validity	Value	From present sample?
States Zalon (1999) demonstrated validity and reliability for use with surgical patients but does not provide values	?	?
Cronbach alpha reliability coefficient—does not indicate why there is a range of values—one assumes the instrument has subscales, but this is not indicated	0.90 to 0.95	Yes

b. Measure—Geriatric Depression Scale

Type of Reliability or Validity	Value	From present sample?
Cronbach alpha reliability coefficient No information on subscales	0.61–0.77	Yes

c. Measure—Modified Fatigue Symptom Checklist

Type of Reliability or Validity	Value	From present sample?
States the reliability and validity of the MFSC has been established in different clinical populations, including the elderly However, no information on values provided Cronbach alpha reliability coefficient	0.87–0.92	Yes

d. Measure—Enforced Social Dependency Scale

Type of Reliability or Validity	Value	From present sample?
Cronbach alpha reliability coefficient	0.69–0.80	Yes

e. Measure—Self-Perception of Recovery After Surgery

Type of Reliability or Validity	Value	From present sample?

None Reported

Sethares and Elliott's study

a. Measure—Heart Failure Readmission Rates

Type of Reliability or Validity	Value	From present sample?
None Reported		

b. Measure—Minnesota Living with Heart Failure Questionnaire

Type of Reliability or Validity	Value	From present sample?
Construct validity	R = 0.80, p = 0.01	No
Cronbach's alpha on total instrument	0.94	No
Cronbach's alpha on total instrument	0.87	Yes

c. Measure—Health Belief Scales

Type of Reliability or Validity	Value	From present sample?
Benefits of medications subscale	0.87	No
Benefits of medications subscale	0.87	Yes
Barriers of medications subscale	0.91	No
Barriers of medications subscale	0.72	Yes
Benefits of diet subscale	0.84	No
Benefits of diet subscale	0.85	Yes
Barriers of diet subscale	0.69	No
Barriers of diet subscale	0.62	Yes
Benefits of self-monitoring	0.89	Yes
Barriers of self-monitoring	0.83	Yes
Content validity	81% agreement	No
Confirmatory factor analysis—BDCS	41% of variance explained	No
Confirmatory factor analysis—BMCS	50% of variance explained	No

3. Adequacy of each measure:
   a. Zalon's study—The only information provided is reliability information. This information appears to be values of the subscales of all of the instruments. However, the author does not indicate this. If the range of Cronbach alphas are subscale values, most are acceptable values. Total scale reliabilities are not provided. This may be because total score values were not used. There is insufficient information to judge the validity of these instruments. The author indicated that there is evidence of validity but does not report numerical values, which would allow us to assess their validity rather than relying on the author's judgment.
   b. Sethares and Elliott's study—These authors provide excellent information on the reliability and validity of their measurement methods, including values from previous publications and from the current sample. The values indicate that the measures have good reliability and validity.

CHAPTER 16

Relevant Terms

Check the glossary in the back of your text for definitions.

Key Ideas

1. All
2. Self-report
3. Direct
4. Alter the reading
5. Consistency
6. Control; content
7. Higher
8. Depth
9. Precise
10. The Likert scale
11. The visual analogue

12. HAPI (Health and Psychological Instruments) On-line

Making Connections

1. b	6. j	11. l
2. f	7. g	12. c
3. n	8. m	13. e
4. a	9. h	14. d
5. k	10. i	

Puzzles

Word Scramble

In publishing the results of a physiologic study, the measurement technique needs to be described in considerable detail.

Secret Message

Observational categories should be mutually exclusive.

Exercises in Critique

1. Description of measurement method
   Zalon's study
   a. Measure—Pain
      Critique: The Brief Pain Inventory (BPI) was developed by Daut, Cleeland, and Flanery in 1983. The instrument uses numerical scales that range from 0 (no pain) to 10 (pain as bad as you can imagine), severity of pain (worst, least, average, right now) and the interference of pain with daily life (general activity, mood, walking, work, relationships with others, sleep, and enjoyment of life). Two items related to pain relief were not used in the study.
   b. Measure—Depression
      Critique: The Geriatric Depression Scale (GDS-SF) is a 15-item Yes-No checklist developed by Sheikh and Yesavage in 1986. The items are specific to geriatric depression. The short form of the instrument is used; however, the short form is highly correlated with the long form ($r. = 0.84$, $p \leq 0.001$.

c. Measure—Fatigue
Critique: The Modified Fatigue Symptom Checklist (MFSC) was developed by Yoshitake in 1971 and modified by Pugh in 1993. It is a 30-item Likert-type scale with four choices. The scale is measured from a multidimensional perspective and has three subscales: drowsiness, concentration, and physical symptoms.

d. Measure—Functional Status
Critique: The Enforced Social Dependency Scale (ESDS) measures the patient's perspective of the degree of assistance required to perform ordinary activities of daily living, thus indicating how disease and its treatment influence patient responses. The instrument was developed by Benoliel, McCorkle, and Young in 1980. It consists of 10 items in two subscales: personal and social competence. The items in the personal subscale measure the degree of dependence of the patient on others for eating, walking, dressing, traveling, bathing, and toileting using a 6-point scale. The social competence subscale measures activities at home, work, and recreation using a 4-point scale and communication using a 3-point scale. The instrument is administered as a semistructured interview. Scores range from 10 to 51, with higher scores indicating greater dependency.

e. Measure—Self-Perception of Recovery After Surgery
Critique: A 0-100 numerical rating scale is used to measure self perception of recovery after surgery. Participants are asked how much they have recovered from their surgery. This method of measurement has been widely used by the National Center for Health Statistics.

Sethares and Elliott's study

a. Measure—Heart Failure Readmission Rates
Critique: This rate was calculated by counting the total number of admissions for heart failure in each group during the 3-month study interval divided by the number of patients in the group. Each admission was counted as 1 regardless of the number of days the patient was in the hospital.

b. Measure—Ways of Coping Quality of Life
Critique: Minnesota Living with Health Failure (MLHF) questionnaire. Patients with heart failure rate their perception of the extent to which heart failure affects socioeconomic, psychologic, and physical aspects of their daily life, using a rating scale of 0 (not at all) to 5 (very much). Scores range from 0 to 105, with higher scores indicating a worse perceived quality of life.

c. Measure—Benefits and Barriers
Critique: The Health Beliefs Scale was developed by Bennett and colleagues in 1987. The instrument contains three scales based on the Health Beliefs Model: Beliefs about Diet Compliance Scale (12 items), Beliefs About Medication Compliance Scale (12 items), and Beliefs About Self-Monitoring Compliance (18 items), for a total of 42 items. Each scale has two subscales, one of benefits and the other of barriers. The instrument uses Likert-type scale scores from 1 to 5, with 1 being "strongly disagree" and 5 "strongly agree." The benefit subscale and the barrier subscale are scored for each of the three scales

CHAPTER 17

Relevant Terms

Check the glossary in the back of your text for definitions.

Key Ideas

1. Decision points
   a. Whether potential subjects meet the sampling criteria
   b. Whether a subject understands the information needed to give informed consent
   c. What group the subject will be assigned to
   d. Whether the subject comprehends instructions related to providing data
   e. Whether the subject has provided all of the data needed
2. Situations affecting data collection consistency
   a. Using more than one data collector
   b. Variation in days and hours of data collection
   c. Care recently received or currently being received
   d. Experience of data collectors
3. Direct costs of data collection
   a. Purchase of measurement instruments
   b. Typing and duplication of data collection forms
   c. Printing costs
   d. Postage costs
   e. Charges for coding and entering data
   f. Statistical consultation
4. Indirect costs of data collection
   a. Costs of traveling to and from data collection sites
   b. Meals eaten out
   c. Researcher's time
   d. Child care while collecting data
5. Tasks of researcher during data collection
   a. Selecting subjects
   b. Collecting data in a consistent way
   c. Maintaining research controls indicated by the study design

d. Protecting study integrity or validity
e. Solving problems that threaten to disrupt the study

Making Connections

1. Age:
   a. The age ranges are not equal.
   b. There is no category for the age of 18.
   c. The age 45 could be placed in either of two categories (or both).
2. Problems with data coding
   a. Family members with flu:
      • One item cannot be used to code this data because subjects could mark several family members. This would require a separate item for each family member, with each member having a code of 0 = no or 1 = yes.
      • The accuracy of the responses may also be a problem since the individual may not know whether some of these family members had the flu last year and may guess. Leaving a response blank is treated the same as a response of "no" but the subject may have left it blank because the answer is unknown.
      • A subject could have more than one of certain relatives, leaving the subject confused about how to respond. For example, a subject may have two children, one of whom had the flu and the other who did not.
   b. Drugs
      • The number of drugs needing to be coded could be large.
      • The dosage matched with the drug would require a separate data item for each dosage and drug combined.
      • In most studies, there is no useful information emerging from such data because of the large number of categories.
   c. Hospital admission
      • There is a problem with determining what a *day* is in this case. Is a day of

admission 24 hours? If so, when does the day begin and end?
- If the patient is admitted for 36 hours or 60 hours, how many days would this be considered?
- Are the number of days determined consistently, or are the number of days determined somewhat arbitrarily and entered into a database?
- Is the time of admission determined consistently?

d. Voting
- Subjects are likely to respond inconsistently to this form or response set. For example, some subjects might mark Yes with a check before the Yes, whereas others might mark Yes by a check after the Yes. There would be no way to determine later what the subject's intent had been. This could increase the error rate of data collection.

Puzzles

Word Scramble

Problems can be perceived either as a frustration or as a challenge.

Secret Message

If anything can go wrong, it will, and at the worst possible time.

Crossword Puzzle

Across
1. Serendipity
4. Codebook
6. Cleaning data
7. Mortality
8. Computerized database
9. Data coding sheet

Down
2. Data collection plan
3. Coding
5. Data collection

Exercise in Critique

1. Zalon's study: Study examined the recovery process after abdominal surgery. Potential subjects were identified from surgical records. Nurses caring for the patients were then interviewed to determine whether the patients were medically unstable or had experienced episodes of delirium in the preceding 24 hours. Patients were first approached postoperatively to allow inclusion of participants who had undergone emergency surgery. After obtaining consent and ensuring that the participant was resting comfortably, an initial interview was performed or arranged for later at a mutually agreeable time. The Mini-Mental State Examination was used as a screening tool to assess cognitive status. Those with a score less than 24, indicating cognitive impairment, were excluded from the study. During the interview, the Brief Pain Inventory, the Geriatric Depression Scale, the Modified Fatigue Symptom Checklist, the Enforced Social Dependency Scale, and the Self-Perception of Recovery After Surgery rating scale were administered. Demographic and related chart data were obtained at that time. Subjects were given a copy of the consent form, a tentative interview schedule, and contact information. A copy of the instruments were also provided. Participants were contacted by phone 3-5 days after discharge, and at 1 month and 3 months after discharge. During the telephone interviews, the Brief Pain Inventory, the Geriatric Depression Scale, the Modified Fatigue Symptom Checklist, the Enforced Social Dependency Scale, and the Self-Perception of Recovery After Surgery rating scale were administered. Subjects who were rehospitalized were not included in subsequent interviews.

2. Sethares and Elliott's study: Two baccalaureate-prepared research nurses enrolled participants, completed the study intervention as outlined in a detailed protocol, and collected data. Hospitalized subjects whose heart failure had been stabilized were invited to participate in the study. After consent was obtained and subjects were randomly assigned to groups, an interview was conducted to complete the Minnesota Living with Heart Failure questionnaire and to collect demographic data. Subjects in the treatment group were interviewed using the Health Belief Scales to determine areas in which teaching was needed. Additional demographic and medication data were obtained from the medical record and computerized hospital databases. A follow-up visit was made to subjects in the treatment group 7-10 days after discharge. Subjects completed the Health Belief Scales. Medication lists were reviewed, and any medication changes were noted. A final follow-up visit was made to treatment subjects 1 month after discharge. Quality of Life scores were determined, and medications were reviewed for any changes. A telephone call was made to the control subjects by a blinded data collector at 1 month to determine Quality of Life scores using the Minnesota Living with Heart Failure questionnaire.

CHAPTER 18

Relevant Terms

Check the glossary in the back of your text for definitions.

Key Ideas

1. Purposes for statistics
   a. Summarize demographic and study variables
   b. Explore the meaning of deviations in the data

   c. Compare or contrast descriptively
   d. Test the proposed relationships in a theoretical model
   e. Infer that the findings from the sample are indicative of the entire population
   f. Predict
   g. Infer from the sample to a theoretical model
   h. Examine reliability and validity of measurement methods
2. Data analysis steps
   a. Preparation of the data for analysis
   b. Description of the sample
   c. Testing the reliability of measurement
   d. Exploratory analysis of the data
   e. Confirmatory analyses guided by the hypotheses, questions, or objectives
   f. Post hoc analyses
3. Activities of data cleaning
   a. Every datum is cross-checked with the original datum for accuracy.
   b. All identified errors are corrected.
   c. Missing points are identified.
   d. Missing data are entered into the data file.

Making Connections

Terms

1. g	4. e	7. i
2. h	5. f	8. b
3. d	6. c	9. a

Categories

1. c	4. a	6. b
2. d	5. c	7. b
3. a		

Significance

1. b
2. a
3. b

Puzzles

Word Scramble

To be useful, the evidence from data analysis must be carefully examined, organized, and given meaning.

Secret Message

Researchers can never prove things.

Crossword Puzzle

Across

2. Clinical significance
4. Level of significance
6. Platykurtic
8. Power analysis
10. Normal curve
13. Tails
15. Skewed
16. Generalize
18. Transform
19. Leptokurtic
20. Distribution
22. Sampling error
23. Post hoc analysis
24. Symmetry

Down

1. Relationship
3. Infer
5. Probability theory
7. Kurtosis
9. Degrees of freedom
11. Mesokurtic
12. Statistic
14. Parameter
17. Exploratory
21. Bimodal

CHAPTER 19

Relevant Terms

Check the glossary in the back of your text for definitions.

Key Ideas

1. Descriptive
2. Frequency distributions
3. Ungrouped frequency distributions
4. Loss of information
5. Percentage distributions
6. Measures of dispersion
7. Square them
8. Standard deviation
9. Standardized scores
10. Confidence intervals
11. Exploratory data analysis
12. Stem-and-leaf display
13. Residuals
14. Scatter plot
15. Sample description:
    a. Estimates of central tendency are calculated for variables relevant to describing the sample.
    b. Estimates of dispersion are calculated for variables relevant to describing the sample.
    c. Data are examined on each variable using measures of central tendency and dispersion to determine variation in the data and to identify outliers.
    d. Relationships among variables relevant to the sample are examined.
    e. Differences between groups are examined to demonstrate equivalence of study groups.

Making Connections

Significant Differences

1. Partial-Bed-Rest group distribution

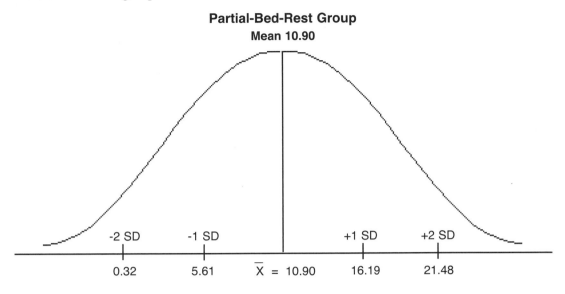

2. Complete-Bed-Rest group distribution

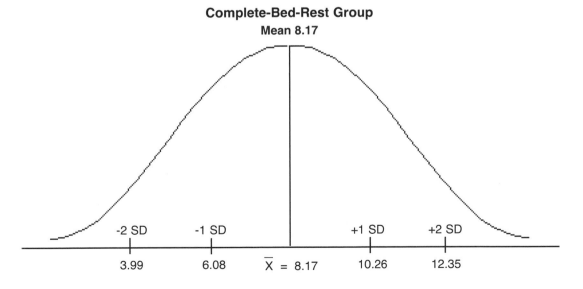

Puzzles

Word Scramble

Using measures of central tendency to describe the nature of the data obscures the impact of extreme values or of deviations in the data.

Secret Message

Data analysis begins with descriptive statistics in any study in which the data are numeric, including some qualitative studies.

Crossword Puzzle

Across	Down
1. Outside	2. Standard deviation
3. Measurement error	4. Stationarity
8. Mean	5. Box-and-whisker plots
11. Outliers	6. Exploratory data analysis
14. Mode	7. Inherent variability
17. Survival analysis	9. Q plot
21. Fence	10. Median
22. Frequencies	12. Forecasting
23. Noise	13. Ungrouped frequency
24. Pattern	15. Difference score
25. Dispersion	16. Far out
26. Residual analysis	18. Scatter plots
	19. Sum of squares
	20. Hinges

Exercises in Critique

1. Zalon reports the number of subjects who met the criteria, the number who refused to participate, and the number who were missed. Information was provided on the following demographic characteristics of the sample: age, gender, ethnicity, education, type of surgery, average length of hospital stay, employment status, marital status, and the presence of chronic painful conditions. Table 1 provides descriptive data on each of the variables, including changes at each measurement point. These changes are also discussed in the text. Reliability values of study instruments in the present sample are reported in the measurement section.

2. Sethares and Elliott describe the sample size, the number originally recruited, the number who withdrew, and the number who died before the study was completed. A t test was run to compare variable values of subjects who died with those who completed the study. No significant differences were found. Demographic characteristics are presented in Tables 1 and 2. Comparisons of the treatment group and the control group revealed no significant differences. Reliability data are provided on measures used in the study. The authors also report the following discussion of preliminary analyses in their study: "Descriptive statistics were computed on all study variables and examined for the presence of random or systematic missing data, significant skewness, and outliers. Appropriate reliability and validity measures were performed on measurement instruments. Because the outcome variable of HF readmission rates was skewed, the nonparametric Kruskal-Wallis statistic was computed to determine differences in HF readmission rates between the treatment and control groups. The benefits, barriers, and quality of life data were not skewed" (p. 255).

CHAPTER 20

Relevant Terms

Check the glossary in the back of your text for definitions.

Key Ideas

1. Relationships
2. One
3. Full range
4. Regression line
5. High; low
6. Interval
7. Phi, contingency coefficient, Cramer's V, or lambda
8. Positive or negative; magnitude or strength
9. ranked
10. Correlational matrix
11. Spurious
12. Factor analysis
13. Two, two
14. Theories

Making Connections

Terms

1. o	7. g	13. m
2. c	8. p	14. n
3. l	9. i	15. h
4. a	10. j	16. d
5. r	11. k	17. a
6. f	12. b	18. e

McNee and McCabe (2004)

$r = 0.37$ M
$r = 0.32$ M
$r = 0.46$ M

Gary and Yarandi (2004)

1. Two factors were identified. The first factor included items describing negative feelings, and the author named it the cognitive dimension. The second factor included items describing physical symptoms. This factor was named the somatic-affective domain. The amount of variation in responses to items in the scale explained by the two factors was 89%. The two factors are correlated with $r = 0.57$.

Puzzles

Word Scramble

Weak correlations may be important when combined with other variables.

Secret Message

In preparation for correlational analysis, data collection strategies should be planned to maximize the possibility of obtaining the full range of possible values on each variable to be used in the analysis.

Crossword Puzzle

Across	Down
1. Scatter diagram	2. Goodness of fit
5. Factor rotation	3. Curvilinear relation
6. Strength	4. Eigenvalues
7. Factor loading	6. Scree test
10. Spurious	8. Positive linear
14. Exogenous	9. Path coefficient
15. Factor	11. Oblique rotation
17. Latent	12. Regression line
18. Weak	13. Endogenous
19. Loading	16. Canonical
20. Homoscedastic	
21. Bivariate	
22. Residual	
23. Weighting	

CHAPTER 21

Relevant Terms

Check the glossary in the back of your text for definitions.

Key Ideas

1. Variance
2. Probability
3. Causal

4. Independent; dependent
5. x (independent variable); y (dependent variable)
6. Method of least squares
7. R
8. Variance
9. Estimate
10. Analysis of variance (ANOVA)
11. Independent
12. Independent
13. Generalizability
14. Inflated
15. Mixture
16. Predictive equation
17. Group membership
18. Linear discriminant functions (LDFs)

Making Connections

Regression Analysis

1. a. The presence of homoscedasticity equals scatter of values of y above and below the regression line at each value of x (constant variance).
   b. The dependent variable is measured at the interval level.
   c. The expected value of the residual error is zero.
2. $Y = a + bx$
3. a. Dummy variables
   b. Multiplicative terms
   c. Transformed terms
   d. Interval level
4. a. Forward stepwise regression
   b. Backward regression
   c. Simultaneous regression
   d. Hierarchical regression
   e. Logistic regression

Matching

1. l	6. n	11. i
2. j	7. g	12. d
3. c	8. a	13. m
4. h	9. b	14. e
5. k	10. f	15. o

Puzzles

Word Scramble

The goal of regression analysis is to determine how accurately one can predict the value of a dependent variable based on the value or values of one or more independent variables.

Secret Message

Discriminant analysis is designed to determine how accurately one can predict the value or values of one or more independent variables.

Crossword Puzzle

Across
2. Simultaneous regression
3. Predictor variable
5. Predictive validity
10. Discriminant analysis
15. Dummy variables
17. Horizontal axis
18. Cross validation

Down
1. Multiple regression
2. Slope
4. Logistic regression
6. Vertical axis
7. Line of best fit
8. Multiplicative term
9. Discriminant function
11. Hold out sample
12. Homoscedasticity
13. Coefficient R
14. Bivariate
16. Y intercept

Exercises in Critique

1.

Variable	**Level of Measurement**
Pain	Interval
Depression	Ordinal treated as interval
Fatigue	Ordinal treated as interval
Functional status	Ordinal treated as interval
Self-perception of recovery	Interval

Total scores from depression, fatigue, and functional status scales were used for analysis.

2. "Diagnostics conducted for each of the multiple regression analyses indicated that multicollinearity was not a problem."
3. Simultaneous regression
4. Seven regressions were performed because data were collected across three time periods and two dependent variables (functional status and self-perception of recovery) were examined, one at a time. Functional status was predicted at three time periods using pain, depression, and fatigue, and self-perception of recovery was predicted at four time periods using pain, depression, and fatigue.
5. (1) Initial patient encounter. Pain, depression, and fatigue significantly accounted for 5.6% of the variation in self-perception of recovery.
   (2) 3-5 days after discharge. Pain, depression, and fatigue significantly accounted for 13.4% of the variation in functional status. Pain, depression, and fatigue significantly accounted for 12.3% of the variation in self-perception of recovery.
   (3) 1 month after discharge. Pain, depression, and fatigue accounted for 30.8% of the variation in functional status. Pain, depression, and fatigue significantly accounted for 33.2% of the variation in self-perception of recovery.
   (4) 3 months after discharge. Pain, depression, and fatigue significantly contributed to 29.1% of the variation in functional status. Pain, depression, and fatigue significantly accounted for 16.1% of the variation in self-perception of recovery.
6. a. Significant and predicted

CHAPTER 22

Relevant Terms

Check the glossary in the back of your text for definitions.

Key Ideas

1. Independent
2. Dependent
3. Contingency tables
4. Only one entry
5. Robust
6. Within; between
7. Size of the group
8. Regression analysis

Puzzles

Word Scramble

The t-test can be used only one time during analysis to examine data from two samples in a study.

Secret Message

In many cases bivariate analysis does not provide a clear picture of the dynamics in the situation.

Crossword Puzzle

Across
1. Statistic
5. Decision theory
8. Significant
11. Power
12. Omit
14. Regression
15. ANOVA
16. Dependent
17. Causal
18. Mean
19. Tail
20. Variance
21. Range
22. Outliers
23. Median
24. Result
25. Inference

Down
2. t-test
3. Explanatory
4. Mode
5. Distribution
6. Representative
7. Implications
9. Normal curve
10. Chi square
13. Post hoc

Exercises in Critique

1. **Variable**   **Level of Measurement**
   Heart failure   Interval
   Readmission
      rate
2. a. Intervention group
   b. Control group
3. These two groups are independent. Subjects randomly assigned to groups.
4. Kruskall-Wallis one-way analysis of variance by ranks
5. The data were skewed.
6. Because the data were interval but skewed. Since the data were not normally distributed, the best option was Kruskall-Wallace, a nonparametric test that makes no assumptions about the type of distribution. Or Mann-Witney could be used to analyze data.
7. Results: "HF readmission rate was not significantly related to group assignment in this study (p. = .22) As seen in Table IV, 12 subjects in the control group were rehospitalized 1 or more times whereas 6 subjects in the treatment group were rehospitalized 1 or more times." Clearly, there was a difference, but because of the small sample size (70 subjects) the study did not have sufficient power to detect a statistical difference if there actually is one in the real world. One can reasonably question whether this finding is a Type II error. The authors state that "the sample size of 70 for the readmission and quality of life variables was determined through a power analysis with an effect size of 0.35, an alpha of .05, and a power of 0.80." This is a medium effect size. Power analysis would have required a sample of 192 subject to have the capacity to identify a small effect. Polit has shown that most nursing intervention tests require the power to test small effect sizes because of crude measures. One of the reasons identified for Type II errors is a small difference in the measured effect, which may be due to a number of factors, including large varia-

tion in scores on the dependent variable within groups, and/or crude instrumentation that does not measure with precision. See discussion on p. 451. One can also question whether a small effect in this clinical situation would be clinically significant. See discussion p. 452. The costs of readmissions are high, and continued work to refine this intervention could have important effects. One wonders whether work on the intervention is continuing or has been abandoned because of this negative finding. One also wonders what would have happened if the study had been conducted with 192 subjects.

8. b (Nonsignificant)
9. **Variable**   **Level of Measurement**
   Quality of life   Ordinal treated as interval
10. a. Intervention group
    b. Control group
11. The groups are independent
12. Repeated measures ANOVA
13. To compare the quality of life data scores at baseline and 1 month between the treatment and control groups
14. The algorithms do not include tests in which repeated measures are used. Without the repeated measures, the pooled t-test or ANOVA could have been used. The repeated measures ANOVA was developed specifically for this type of data.
15. "For within-subjects effects, there were significant differences in quality-of-life measures at the 2 time points (F = 35.44, p = .000), with both groups reporting improved quality of life at 1 month as expected with a group recruited during hospitalization. The mean quality of life score was 55.5 at baseline and 41.6 at 1 month. The assumption of homogeneity of variance for between-subjects factors was met. There were no significant differences between the group receiving the tailored message intervention and the control group in reported quality of life (F = 1.031, p = .309). The control group had a mean score of 50.9, and the treatment

group had a mean score of 46.2. There was no significant interaction between quality of life and group assigned (F = .217, p = .575)."
16. b (Nonsignificant)
17. Intervention subjects would report fewer barriers and more benefits to performing self-care of HF after receiving the tailored message intervention.

Variable	Level of Measurement
Benefits of medications	Ordinal treated as interval
Benefits of diet	Ordinal treated as interval
Benefits of self-monitoring	Ordinal treated as interval
Barriers of medication	Ordinal treated as interval
Barriers of diet	Ordinal treated as interval
Barriers of self-monitoring	Ordinal treated as interval

18. a. Intervention group at baseline
    b. Intervention group at 1 week
    c. Intervention group at 1 month
19. Groups are dependent.
20. Within-subjects repeated measures ANOVA
21. This procedure was developed specifically for such designs.
22. The procedure is appropriate.
23. "The benefits of medications scores did not change significantly during the study (p = .259). Barriers of medication scores decreased from baseline to the 1 point (p = .000) and significantly decreased from baseline to the 1 month point (p = .000). Benefits of diet significantly increased from baseline to one week (p = .000) and from baseline to one month (p = .000). The barriers of diet significantly decreased from baseline to 1 week (p = .000) and from baseline to 1 month (p = .001). The benefits of self-monitoring significantly improved from baseline to 1 week (p. .000) and from baseline to 1 month (p = .000). Barriers of self-monitoring decreased significantly from baseline to 1 week (p = .002) with further decreases at 1 month."
24. c   Significant and predicted

CHAPTER 23

Relevant Terms
Check the glossary in the back of your text for definitions

Key Ideas
1. Simultaneously with
2. Words; numbers
3. Concreteness; abstraction
4. Decision rules
5. Personality
6. Theorizing
7. Participants
8. Researcher-participant relationships:
   a. Complete participation
   b. Participant-as-observer
   c. Observer-as-participant
   d. Complete observer
9. Characteristics of researcher-participant relationships in qualitative research:
   a. The researcher influences the individuals being studied and, in turn, is influenced by them.
   b. The mere presence of the researcher may alter behavior in the setting.
   c. The researcher's personality is a key factor in conducting the study.
   d. The researcher needs to become closely involved in the subject's experience in order to interpret it.
   e. It is necessary for the researcher to be open to the perceptions of the participants, rather than to attach his or her own meaning to the experience.
   f. Individuals being studied often participate in determining research questions, guiding data collection, and interpreting results.
10. Methods of reducing data in qualitative research:
    a. Coding-developing categories
    b. Reflective remarks
    c. Marginal remarks
    d. Memoing
    e. Developing propositions

11. Methods of drawing conclusions:
    a. Counting
    b. Noting patterns and themes
    c. Seeing plausibility
    d. Clustering
    e. Making metaphors
    f. Splitting variables
    g. Subsuming particulars into the general
    h. Factoring
    i. Noting relations between variables
    j. Finding intervening variables
    k. Building a logical chain of evidence
    l. Making conceptual and theoretical coherence

Making Connections

1. e	7. c	13. f
2. f	8. d	14. d
3. b	9. a	15. a
4. a	10. b	16. c
5. d	11. c	17. e
6. b	12. e	

Puzzles

Word Scramble

Analysis requires cross-checking each bit of data with all the other bits of data.

Secret Message

One important difference between quantitative and qualitative research is the nature of relationships between the researcher and the individuals being studied.

Crossword Puzzle

Across
2. Interpretation
5. Cognitive mapping
9. Segmentation
11. Case study
12. Story
14. Intuiting
15. Data reducing

Down
1. Reflexivity
3. Premature parsimony
4. Story telling
6. Themes
7. Decision trail
8. Dwelling

Across
16. Bracketing
17. Story taker
18. Memoing
19. Explanatory
20. Auditability
21. Coding

Down
10. Participate
13. Triangulation

Exercises in Critique

1. The philosophical base of the study is phenomenology.
2. The author used Giorgi's method.
3. Giorgi is a phenomenological methodologist. Clearly the author intentionally selected a phenomenological approach to the study.
4. The researcher was consistent in following the methodology.
5. The author's logic was easy to follow.
6. The author's selection of subjects seemed limited to women who were involved in church activities. The findings may be limited to those who have such connections.
7. The information provides some guidance to those working with substance abusing women. Their spirituality needs to be included in the treatment plan.

CHAPTER 24

Relevant Terms

Check the glossary in the back of your text for definitions.

Key Ideas

1. Carefully examined, organized, and given meaning, and both statistical and clinical significance need to be assessed
2. a. Abstract thinking
   b. Introspection
   c. Reasoning
   d. Intuition
   e. Synthesis

f. Mathematical logic
g. Gestalt formation
h. Forecasting
3. Reexamination of the research plan
4. Adequately measured
5. Consistently
6. a. How many errors were made in entering the data into the computer?
   b. How many subjects have missing data that could affect statistical analyses?
   c. Were the analyses accurately calculated?
   d. Were statistical assumptions violated?
   e. Were the statistics used appropriate to the data?
7. Amount of variance in the phenomenon
8. The risk of a Type II error in relation to the nonsignificant results
9. Unexpected results
10. Proves anything
11. Going beyond the data
12. a. Make an important difference in people's lives
   b. Have external validity
   c. Possible to generalize the findings far beyond the study sample so that the findings have the potential to affect large numbers of people
   d. Go beyond concrete facts to abstractions
   e. Lead to the generation of theory or revisions in existing theory
   f. Have implications for one or more disciplines in addition to nursing
13. The study sample
14. Empirical generalizations
15. Many studies
16. Theory

Making Connections

1. c   3. f   5. d
2. a   4. e   6. b

Puzzles

Word Scramble

Evaluating the research process used in the study, producing meaning from the results, and forecasting the usefulness of the findings, all of which are involved in interpretation, require high-level intellectual processes.

Secret Message

To be useful, the evidence from data analysis needs to be carefully examined, organized, and given meaning, and both statistical and clinical significance needs to be examined.

Crossword Puzzle

Across
3. Landmark studies
7. Evidence
9. Conclusion
10. Translate
11. Implications

Down
1. Practical significance
2. Significance
4. Generalization
5. Interpretation
6. Findings
8. Results

Exercises in Critique

1. Findings: Pain, depression, and fatigue are significantly related to functional status as well as self-perception of recovery in older postoperative abdominal surgery patients. Results that contribute to this finding:
   - Multiple regression analysis with the variables entered at once indicates that pain, depression, and fatigue significantly accounted for 13.4% of the variation in functional status during the immediate (3-5 days) postoperative period.
   - At 1 month after discharge, pain, depression, and fatigue accounted for 30.8% of the variation in functional status.
   - At 3 months after discharge, pain, depression, and fatigue significantly accounted for 29.1% of the variation in functional status.

- The results of the multiple regres-sion analysis with the variables entered at once indicate that pain, depression, and fatigue significantly accounted for 5.6% of the variation in self-perception of recovery at the initial measurement during hospital-ization.
- At 3-5 days after discharge, pain, depression, and fatigue significantly accounted for 12.3% of the variation in self-perception of recovery.
- At 1 month after discharge, pain, depression, and fatigue significantly accounted for 33.2% of the variation in self-perception of recovery.
- At 3 months after discharge, pain, depression, and fatighe significantly accounted for 16.1% of the variation in self-perception of recovery.

2. Conclusions: "The results of this investiga-tion are consistent with those of others addressing functional status and illness from a more global perspective as well as findings of studies focusing on pain, depres-sion, and fatigue at all three data collection times."
3. Zalon's conclusions are warranted by the data. In addition, she links them to findings of previous studies.
4. Implications: "This indicates that interven-tions to address pain, depression, and fatigue are important regardless of the rea-son for hospitalization."
5. Evaluation of implications: appropriate to findings
6. Clinical significance: "The proportion of variation explained by pain, depression, and fatigue 1 and 3 months after discharge high-lights the importance of factors that have the potential for effective treatment during the postoperative period. Although pain contributed to the variation in functional status at 1 and 3 months, it should be noted that a number of participants reported that their pain at 3 months was not related to the incision or surgery, but rather to a chronic painful condition. Thus, patients with chronic painful conditions need to have their pain managed well to maximize their recovery from surgery."
7. Generalizations: Home care reimbursement has been limited in recent years. This is evi-dent in that only one third of the study par-ticipants received home care services. Therefore, strategies to facilitate effective pain management after discharge, including the management of chronic pain, need to be addressed in the acute care setting.
8. Suggestions for further studies: "A limita-tion of this study is that baseline data were not available because the participants did not complete the instruments preoperatively. Therefore, additional research including baseline data is recommended to describe the impact of surgery on recovery."

Chapter 25

Relevant Terms

1. d	4. g	7. f
2. b	5. a	8. e
3. h	6. c	9. i

Key Ideas

1. Any four of the following:
   a. Background and significance of the problem and problem statement
   b. Statement of the purpose
   c. Presentation of the literature review, empirical and theoretical literature
   d. Discussion of the framework
   e. Identification of research objectives, questions, or hypotheses (if applicable)
   f. Identification of conceptual and opera-tional definitions of variables
2. a. Discussion of the research design
   b. Description of the sample and setting
   c. Description of the methods of measure-ment
   d. Discussion of the data collection process

e. Description of the intervention and intervention protocol (if appropriate)
3. Methods
4. Data analysis procedures; presentation of results
5. Bar graphs; line graphs
6. Results
7. Do
8. Meta-analyses; power analysis
9. Tables; figures
10. a. Presentation of major findings
    b. Identification of the limitations
    c. Identification of conclusions
    d. Discussion of the implications for nursing practice
    e. Recommendations for further research
11. Framework
12. Implications of the findings for nursing practice
13. a. Entry into the site
    b. Selection of participants
    c. Documentation of ethical considerations
    d. Description of the data collection process
14. a. Identification of the phenomenon to be studied
    b. Identification of the aim or purpose of the study
    c. Identification of the study questions
    d. Identification of the qualitative approach used to conduct the study
    e. Discussion of the significance of the study to nursing
    f. Evolution of the study
15. Theory; model; culture; event; phenomenon
16. Theses; dissertations
17. a. Nurses (clinicians, educators, and researchers)
    b. Other health professionals
    c. Policy makers
    d. Consumers of health care services
18. Clinicians; educators; researchers
19. Internet
20. a. Receiving acceptance as a presenter
    b. Developing a research report
    c. Delivering the report

d. Responding to questions
21. Abstract
22. 5
23. One-to-one
24. a. Basic requirements of the journal
    b. The journal's refereed status
    c. The recent articles published in the journal
25. Query letter
26. a. Acceptance of the manuscript as submitted
    b. Acceptance of the manuscript pending minor revisions
    c. Tentative acceptance of the manuscript pending major revisions
    d. Rejection of the manuscript
27. Poorly written
28. Books; chapters in books
29. Duplicate publications
30. Reference list

Making Connections

1. a	5. c	8. d
2. b	6. a	9. b
3. d	7. c	10. d
4. a		

Exercises in Critique

Sethares and Elliott Study

1. Yes, Sethares and Elliott (2004) cover the main areas of a research report: Introduction, Methods, Results, and Discussion. They also included additional headings that comprise the steps of the research process.
    a. Introduction, Literature Review, Conceptual Framework, Study Purposes and Research Questions, Hypotheses
    b. Methods, Sample, Instruments (heart failure readmission rates; quality of life; benefits and barriers), Procedure, Intervention (treatment subjects; control subjects), Analysis
    c. Results (readmission rates; quality of life; benefits and barriers)
    d. Discussion, Implications

2. This article was published in *Heart & Lung*, a journal read by clinicians in the specialty areas of critical care and medical-surgical nursing. Researchers and educators also read this journal to add to their knowledge base of care provided to patients with complex acute and chronic illnesses. The editor of this journal, Kathleen Stone, is a nurse, and the section editors and executive editorial board are all nurses. The editorial board includes both nurses and physicians. The journal is probably read mainly by nurses and a limited number of other health professionals. This journal is probably not read by many consumers.

Wright Study

1. Yes, Wright (2003) does include most of the main sections of a research report: Introduction provided but not labeled as such; Methods (extensive); Findings; Discussion. No section called Results, but results are covered in the Findings section.
   a. Introduction (provided but not labeled), Purpose
   b. Methods (Philosophical Perspective; Methodology; Methods; Study Participants; Phenomenological Rigor; Procedure and Data Collection)
   c. Findings
   d. Discussion; Limitations; Conclusions and Implications
2. This study was published in *Archives of Psychiatric Nursing*, which is read by clinicians, educators, and researchers with a specialty area in psychiatric nursing. The editor of this journal, Judith Krauss, is a nurse, and the associate editors and editorial board members are all nurses. This journal is probably read mainly by nurses and a limited number of other professionals, such as counselors and psychiatrists, and maybe a few consumers.

Zalon Study

1. Yes, Zalon (2004) includes the four main sections of a research report: Introduction (included but not labeled as such); Research Design and Methods; Results; Discussion.
   a. Introduction (content included but not labeled as such)
   b. Research Design and Methods (Sample; Instruments; Demographic and Medical Record Data; Procedures)
   c. Results
   d. Discussion
2. This study was published in *Nursing Research*, which is read by researchers, educators, and some expert clinicians. The editor of this journal, Molly Dougherty, is a nurse, and the editorial board is also composed of nurses. This journal is probably read mainly by nurses, a limited number of other health professionals, and a few consumers.

CHAPTER 26

Relevant Terms

1. m	6. b	11. l
2. c	7. e	12. f
3. a	8. j	13. k
4. n	9. h	14. i
5. d	10. g	15. o

Key Ideas

1. Strengths; weaknesses; meaning; significance
2. You could include any of the following:
   a. What are the major strengths of the study?
   b. What are the major weaknesses of the study?
   c. Are the findings from the study an accurate reflection of reality?

d. What is the significance of the findings for nursing?

e. Are the findings consistent with those for previous studies?

3. If you are an undergraduate nursing student, you might critique research to share the findings with another health care professional. You might read and critique studies to solve a problem in practice or to summarize research in a topic area for use in practice. You might critique a proposed study to determine whether it is ethical to conduct in your clinical agency. If you are a student in a master's program, you might do all the above listed behaviors and also critique studies to use in developing the literature review section of a research proposal. Thus you would be summarizing the current knowledge base in a selected area as the basis for conducting your own study. If you are a doctoral student, you might conceptually cluster the findings from several studies to determine the current body of knowledge in a selected area to promote evidence-based practice in this area.

4. a. Appropriateness of the study for the program planned
   b. Completeness of the research project
   c. Overall quality of the work
   d. Contribution of the study to nursing scholarship
   e. Contribution of the study to nursing theory
   f. Originality of the work (not previously published)
   g. Clarity and completeness of the abstract

5. a. Examine the expertise of the researchers
   b. Critique the entire study
   c. Address the study's strengths
   d. Address the study's weaknesses
   e. Examine the adequacy of the study's logical links
   f. Evaluate the contribution of the study to nursing knowledge

6. a. Comprehension
   b. Comparison
   c. Analysis
   d. Evaluation
   e. Conceptual clustering

7. a. Descriptive vividness
   b. Methodological congruence
   c. Analytical preciseness
   d. Theoretical connectedness
   e. Heuristic relevance

Exercises in Critique

Conduct the critiques outlined in this section of your study guide. Review the answers for the critique exercises in Chapters 5-11 and Chapters 14-24 to assist you. Also ask your instructor to clarify any questions that you might have and to review your work when done.

CHAPTER 27

Relevant Terms

1. q	9. j	16. a
2. t	10. r	17. s
3. n	11. p	18. e
4. c	12. u	19. o
5. m	13. k	20. l
6. v	14. i	21. b
7. f	15. g	22. h
8. d		

Key Ideas

1. Evidence-based practice promotes desired outcomes for patients, nurses, and health care agencies. Some of these positive outcomes include:
   a. Improved quality of care
   b. Improved patient outcomes such as decreased signs and symptoms, improved functional status, physical and psychological health
   c. Decreased recovery time
   d. Decreased need for health care services
   e. Decreased cost of care
   f. Improved work environment for nurses with increased productivity

g. Increased access to care by providing different types of health care agencies and services by a variety of health care providers

h. Increased patient satisfaction with care

2. Rogers' Theory of Diffusion of Innovations

3. You could identify any of the following:
   a. Research journals
   b. Clinical journals with a major focus on publishing research articles
   c. Evidence-based websites such as the Agency for Healthcare Research and Quality and many others that communicate evidence-based guidelines and reference a variety of research publications
   d. Professional nursing meetings and conferences
   e. Nursing research conferences
   f. Some collaborative groups of nurses and other health professionals that share research findings
   g. Television news reports
   h. Newspapers
   i. Some popular magazines

4. You could identify any of the following:
   a. Axford and Cutchen (1977) developed a preoperative teaching program.
   b. Dracup and Breu (1978) devised a care plan for grieving spouses.
   c. Wichita (1977) developed a program to treat and prevent constipation in nursing home residents.

5. a. Identification and synthesis of multiple studies on a selected topic
   b. Organization of research knowledge into a solution or clinical protocol for practice
   c. Transformation of the clinical protocol into specific nursing actions that are administered to patients
   d. Clinical evaluation of the new practice to determine whether it produced the desired outcome

6. You could identify any of the following:
   a. Previous practice of the agency
   b. Felt needs/problems identified in the agency
   c. Innovativeness of those working in the agency
   d. Norms of the social system within the agency

7. You could identify any of the following:
   a. Structured preoperative teaching
   b. Reducing diarrhea in tube-fed patients
   c. Preoperative sensory preparation to promote recovery
   d. Preventing decubitus ulcers
   e. Intravenous cannula change
   f. Closed urinary drainage systems
   g. Distress reduction through sensory preparation
   h. Mutual goal-setting in patient care
   i. Clean intermittent catheterization
   j. Pain: deliberative nursing interventions

8. a. Research findings barriers
      Examples: limited research conducted for certain clinical problems; studies conducted lack replication; limited communication of research findings; research reports are complex and difficult to read
   b. Barriers created by practicing nurses
      Examples: practicing nurses do not value research; they are unwilling to read research reports; they lack the skills to read research reports
   c. Barriers created by organizations
      Examples: some organizations have traditional leadership that is reluctant to change; organizations do not provide support for making changes based on research

9. a. Relative advantage
   b. Compatibility
   c. Complexity
   d. Trialability
   e. Observability

10. Examining the innovation or change for practice and then deciding not to adopt it

11. That the innovation was never seriously considered for use in practice

12. a. Immediate use—using research-based intervention in practice exactly as it was developed
    b. Reinvention—occurs when the research intervention is modified to meet the needs of a healthcare agency or nurses within the agency
    c. Cognitive change—occurs when nurses incorporate research findings into their knowledge base and use this information to defend a point or to write agency protocols or policies or develop a clinical paper for presentation
13. a. Replacement discontinuance
    b. Disenchantment discontinuance
14. a. Integrative reviews of research (A list of integrative reviews of research is included on the textbook website.)
    b. Meta-analysis (A list of meta-analyses is included on the textbook website.)
15. The phases of the Stetler Model are:
    a. Phase I—Preparation
    b. Phase 11—Validation
    c. Phase III—Comparative Evaluation/Decision-Making
    d. Phase IV—Translation/Application
    e. Phase V—Evaluation
16. Feasibility; current practice
17. a. Use research evidence in practice now.
    b. Consider using research knowledge in practice.
    c. Do not use the research findings in practice.
18. Iowa
19. Evidence-based guidelines
20. Evidence-based practice

Making Connections

Stages

1. e
2. c
3. a
4. d
5. b

Types of Adopters

1. d
2. a
3. e
4. c
5. b

Going Beyond

1. Obtain the answers to these questions by gathering information in the agencies where you have clinical practice this semester. You could also use your work site and answer these questions to determine how rapidly research information might be used in this practice setting.
2. Use the steps of Rogers' Theory of Utilization, Stetler's Model of Research Utilization to Facilitate Evidence-Based Practice, or the Iowa Model of Evidence-Based Practice as outlined in Chapter 27 of your text to assist you in using research knowledge in practice. Seek guidance from your instructor as needed.
3. Use the Grove Model for Implementing Evidence-Based Practice Guidelines in Chapter 27 in your text to implement an evidence-based practice guideline from the Agency for Healthcare Research and Quality (www.ahrq.gov).

CHAPTER 28

Relevant Terms

1. d
2. e
3. c
4. a
5. b

Key Ideas

1. Concise; complete
2. a. Developing ideas logically
   b. Determining the depth or detail of the proposal content
   c. Identifying critical points in the proposal

d. Developing esthetically appealing copy
3. American Psychological Association (APA)
4. a. Introduction
   b. Review of relevant literature
   c. Framework
   d. Methods and procedures
5. a. Describing how the research situation will be structured
   b. Detailing the treatment to be implemented
   c. Describing how the effect of the treatment will be measured
   d. Indicating the variables to be controlled and the methods for controlling them
   e. Identifying uncontrolled extraneous variables and determining their impact on the findings
   f. Describing the methods for assigning subjects to the treatment and control groups
   g. Describing the strengths and weaknesses of a design
6. Institutional research review; IRB
7. You could have identified any of the following aspects of the introduction to a qualitative study:
   a. Identify the phenomenon to be studied
   b. Identify the study aim or purpose
   c. State the study questions
   d. Describe the evolution of the study
   e. Provide a rationale for conducting the study
   f. Place the study in context historically
   g. Discuss the researcher's experience with the phenomenon
   h. Discuss the relevance of the study to nursing
8. a. Letter of transmittal
   b. Brief introduction of the proposed research project
   c. Personnel for the project
   d. Facilities to be used
   e. Budget

9. a. To evaluate the quality of the study
   b. To ensure that adequate measures are being taken to protect human subjects
   c. To evaluate the impact of conducting the study on the reviewing institution
10. a. The use of the clinical facility's name in reporting findings
    b. Presentation and publication of the study
    c. Authorship of publications
11. Representative; funding agency
12. a. What needs to be changed?
    b. Why is the change necessary?
    c. How will the change affect the implementation of the study and the study findings?

Making Connections

1. a
2. a, b
3. a
4. b
5. b

Going Beyond

1. Review the guidelines and example quantitative research proposal presented in Chapter 28. Think about developing the proposal with another student or with a member of a health care agency.
2. Meet with the chair of the institutional review board for the agency where you would like to conduct your study. Follow the guidelines provided to obtain approval to conduct your study in that agency. Review the helpful hints in Chapter 28 to assist you in successfully defending your proposed study.

CHAPTER 29

Relevant Terms

Check the glossary in the back of your text for definitions.

Key Ideas

1. The cost of the study tends to increase
2. Scientific credibility
3. Small grants
4. Focus their efforts in one area of study
5. Initiate a program of research
6. Reviewing proposals and making decisions about funding
7. Small grants
8. Foundation directory
9. The foundation's guidelines
10. The federal government
11. Catalog of Federal Domestic Assistance
12. Contact an official with the government agency early in the planning process to inform the agency of the intent to submit a proposal
13. Federal Register
14. Highly competitive
15. Not only identifies the problem of concern but also describes the design of the study
16. A study section
17. 1 year
18. Before the first grant is ended
19. Strategies used to gain skills in grantsmanship:
    a. Attend grantsmanship courses
    b. Develop a reference group
    c. Join research organizations
    d. Serve on research committees
    e. Network
    f. Assist a researcher
    g. Obtain a mentor
20. Sources of small grant funding:
    a. Within the university
    b. Nursing organizations
    c. Sigma Theta Tau
    d. Local agencies
    e. Private individuals

Puzzles

Word Scramble

Well-designed studies can be expensive.

Secret Message

The scientific credibility of the profession is related to the quality of studies conducted by its researchers.

Crossword Puzzle

Across
1. Funded research
6. Pink sheet
8. Mentor
9. Requests for proposals
10. Grantsmanship
11. Research grant
12. Request for application

Down
2. Reference group
3. Networking
4. Foundation grant
5. Developmental grant
7. Query letter

The effect of a tailored message intervention on heart failure readmission rates, quality of life, and benefit and barrier beliefs in persons with heart failure

KRISTEN A. SETHARES, RN, PhD, AND
KATHLEEN ELLIOTT, BN, MSN, ANP-C, DARTMOUTH, MASSACHUSETTS

Objective: The purpose of this study was to determine the effect of a tailored message intervention on heart failure readmission rates, quality of life, and health beliefs in persons with heart failure (HF).

Design: This randomized control trial provided a tailored message intervention during hospitalization and 1 week and 1 month after discharge.

Theoretic Framework: The organizing framework was the Health Belief Model.

Subjects: Seventy persons with a primary diagnosis of chronic HF were included in the study.

Results: HF readmission rates and quality of life did not significantly differ between the treatment and control groups. Health beliefs, except for benefits of medications, significantly changed from baseline in the treatment group in directions posited by the Health Belief Model.

Conclusions: A tailored message intervention changed the beliefs of the person with HF in regard to the benefits and barriers of taking medications, following a sodium-restricted diet, and self-monitoring for signs of fluid overload. Future research is needed to explore the effect of health belief changes on actual self-care behaviors. (Heart Lung © 2004; 33:249-60.)

From Sethares, K.A., & Elliott, K. (2004). The effect of a tailored message intervention on heart failure readmission rates, quality of life, and benefit and barrier beliefs in persons with heart failure. Heart & Lung, 33(4), 249-260. © 2003 Elsevier Inc. All rights reserved.

INTRODUCTION

Cardiovascular disease, the leading cause of death in the United States today, is one of the most prevalent chronic illnesses of adulthood.[1] A common clinical endpoint of many cardiovascular disorders is heart failure (HF), defined as the inability of the heart to provide the tissues with oxygen at a rate necessary to meet oxidative requirements.[2] The American College of Cardiology/American Heart Association Task Force reports that 4.8 million Americans experience HF, with 550,000 new cases and 50,000 deaths reported annually.[1,3] In 1999, 962,000 Americans were discharged from acute care facilities with a primary diagnosis of HF, the most prevalent diagnosis in those aged more than 65 years.

HF is characterized by an unstable course of illness with unpredictable exacerbations and progression of symptoms, often without further damage to the myocardium.[4] Symptoms such as weight gain, edema, dyspnea, and fatigue characterize these exacerbations and further limit functional status and quality of life.[5,6] Because HF is a chronic condition, most lifestyle change is made on an outpatient basis, necessitating follow-up in the home setting to evaluate medication effectiveness, monitor symptoms, and promote self-care behaviors. However, current capitation rates fiscally limit the quantity of nursing care provided in the home. The end result of these combined factors is a high cost, reported to be close to 10 billion dollars.[7]

It is imperative that nurses develop innovative methods to improve the self-care behaviors of this population while attempting to decrease costly rehospitalizations. A tailored message intervention is one proposed alternative. In this case, education is based on an evaluation of the beliefs of the person with HF concerning perceived benefits and perceived barriers of performing certain HF self-care behaviors. In self-care areas with more identified barriers or less perceived benefits, a tailored message is given. The purpose of this investigation was to determine whether the tailored message intervention decreased readmission rates, improved reported quality of life, and changed beliefs about perceived benefits and perceived barriers of self-care in persons with HF.

LITERATURE REVIEW

Research demonstrates that older adults with HF have the highest hospital readmission rates, ranging from 29% to 47% of all hospitalized adult patient groups, primarily in the first few weeks after discharge.[8–11] As a result, most intervention studies have focused on trying to decrease readmission rates in this vulnerable population. Interdisciplinary teams composed of dietitians, social workers, pharmacists, physicians, and nurses have all played a role in significantly reducing readmission rates of persons with HF through education, discharge planning, and medication evaluation.[12–14] Standardized care maps guided the interdisciplinary team efforts in several studies.[4,15–17] Disease management interventions that include monitoring across the spectrum of care by multidisciplinary teams seek to improve the management of HF through guideline-based surveillance, education, and frequent outpatient follow-up.[15–20] These plans have shown moderate success in decreasing readmission rates and costs in a subset of the population with HF. However, this type of plan fails to account for the activity limitations of some persons with HF and the difficulty of attending frequent outpatient visits because of symptoms brought on by minimal activity. Anderson et al[8] and Elkman et al[21] reported that 29% to 50% of persons with HF have difficulty attending outpatient follow-up appointments because of symptoms during activity that limit function.

Numerous interventions have included some component of telephone follow-up for persons with HF, resulting in reduced readmission rates,[22,23] no change,[21] and significantly increased readmission rates.[24] Although these interventions minimize the need for frequent outpatient follow-up, nurses still managed the care of HF. In most cases, the telephone follow-up was provided by nurses, using standardized algorithms that assessed symptoms and self-care behaviors.[23,25] Follow-up was performed in cases in which persons reported increased symptoms. In these models of care, the frequent follow-up provided by nurses did not allow the person with HF to develop his or her own ability to initiate follow-up for identified symptoms.

Transitional care models, first described by Brooten and colleagues[26] for low birth weight infants, have also been applied to elderly persons with HF. In this model, advance practice nurses assisted persons with cardiac diagnoses to transition from the hospital to home by providing individualized discharge planning, education, and follow-up for the first 2 weeks at home.[14,27–29] Most of the interventions provided by the advance practice nurses included surveillance of signs and symptoms and health teaching.[30] The use of this model has resulted in significant reductions in readmission rates, cost, and length of time to readmission. However, not all regions of the country have advanced practice nurses with the knowledge and skills necessary to provide these services.

In many of these studies, the efficacy of the educational component of the intervention alone has been less well studied. In those studies that did contain educational interventions, standardized forms and care maps guided the education. Teaching interventions based on clinical guidelines and care maps alone fail to account for the individual characteristics present in the learner.[31–36] Nurses educating persons with HF need to include individualized learning assessments in all plans of care to account for multiple contextual variables present in these individuals. Transfer of knowledge alone is often not sufficient to promote behavior change without some further behavioral support strategies throughout the process, often in the outpatient setting.[37,38] Further, the Joint Commission on Accreditation of Healthcare Organization[39] mandates that individuals must receive education at a level appro-

priate to their degree of understanding. Nurses are well suited to provide this education because of their knowledge and close interpersonal relationship with persons with HF. The use of a tailored message intervention may reduce the need for reading if the education is verbal and tailored to the specific learning needs of the person with HF.

CONCEPTUAL FRAMEWORK

The Health Belief Model (HBM) provides the organizing framework for the study. In this model, an individual performs a health behavior based on perceived susceptibility, perceived severity, perceived benefits, and perceived barriers to an illness.[40–42] Perceived susceptibility and perceived severity relate to the psychologic components of the model whereby individuals evaluate subjective risk of HF to them. Inherent in the process of psychologic evaluation of risk is both internal moderating factors and external cues to action. Personal factors, including demographics, sociocultural variables, and level of knowledge about HF, are believed to modify the health beliefs of persons with HF.[40] Unlike demographic and sociocultural variables that are stable traits of persons, knowledge is amenable to change. External cues to action are found in the mass media and through contact with health care providers.[43] Severity of illness in the person with HF may be manifest in potentially function-limiting symptoms, such as shortness of breath and fatigue.

Perceived benefits of performing a certain health behavior relate to a subjectively determined course of action that reduces the susceptibility of illness.[40] Kasl[44] reconceptualized susceptibility for chronically ill persons as resusceptibility to exacerbations of the illness. In the case of the person with HF, taking medications or following a low-salt diet may reduce the progression of symptoms and be seen as beneficial. These benefits are weighed against perceived barriers to a certain course of action. Perceived barriers are the potential negative consequences of a certain health behavior. In the population with HF, a barrier to following medication recommendations might be the outcome of frequent urination caused by diuretic therapy. In this case, the person with HF would weigh risks and benefits before making a decision about whether to follow a recommended course of action.

In this study, the tailored message intervention focused on decreasing client-identified barriers to self-care. Individualized teaching by a nurse focused on enhancing the benefits and decreasing the barriers to self-care of a person with HF. Although a person with HF may believe that a certain behavior will decrease HF symptoms, if that action is expensive, time-consuming, or unpleasant, these can serve as barriers to taking that action. If readiness to act is high and barriers to act are low, then self-care action is more likely.[45] The goal of this tailored message intervention was to improve the readiness of the person with HF to perform self-care behaviors by decreasing identified barriers and increasing perceived benefits of action while supporting the individual needs of the person with HF in the process. By changing perceived beliefs related to self-care, it is anticipated that persons with HF will improve self-care behaviors, which may lead to improved quality of life and lower readmission rates.

STUDY PURPOSES AND RESEARCH QUESTIONS

This study determines the efficacy of a tailored message intervention administered during hospital admission and at 1 week and 1 month after discharge on HF readmission rates, reported quality of life, and perceived benefit and barrier beliefs in elderly patients with HF. The times selected for study correspond with times identified in the literature as the period of greatest risk for rehospitalization in elderly patients.[8,27,28] The following research questions are the basis for the study:

1. Do individuals who receive the tailored message intervention have lower HF readmission rates than a control group at 3 months?
2. Do individuals who receive a tailored message intervention report better quality of life at baseline and 1 month after discharge than a control group?
3. What is the effect of the tailored message intervention on the perceived benefit and barrier beliefs of the treatment group at baseline, 1 week, and 1 month?

HYPOTHESES

There were 3 hypotheses for the study. The first 2 hypotheses were that persons who received the intervention would have lower HF readmission rates and report better quality of life. The third hypothesis was that intervention subjects would report fewer barriers and more benefits to performing self-care of HF after receiving the tailored message intervention.

METHODS

A randomized control trial was used to evaluate the effect of a tailored message intervention on HF readmission rates, quality of life, and perceived benefit and barrier beliefs in an elderly sample of subjects with HF. Benefit and barrier scores were measured during initial hospitalization and 1 week and 1 month after discharge in the treatment group. Quality of life scores were obtained in both groups during initial hospitalization and 1 month after hospital discharge. HF readmission rates were measured 3 months after hospital discharge in both groups.

SAMPLE

The sample was drawn from a population of adults with a primary diagnosis of chronic HF who were admitted to 1 community hospital in the Northeast between October 1999 and December 2000. Persons with HF who consented to participate were randomly assigned to the treatment or control group. Criteria for study enrollment included the following: (1) primary diagnosis of either systolic or diastolic HF listed in the medical record, confirmed by the presence of symptoms of HF for 3 months or longer; (2) echocardiography for confirmation of ejection fraction; (3) English speaking; (4) freedom from serious cognitive deficits, as determined by the Mini Mental Status Exam; and (5) anticipated return to a community setting, rather than long-term care. HF stage (New York Heart Association [NYHA]) was determined by asking the subject the current level of activity that precipitated symptoms. The sample size of 70 for the readmission and quality of life variables was determined through a power analysis with an effect size of 0.35, an alpha of .05, and a power of 0.80.[46]

Data were collected by a baccalaureate-prepared research nurse during an interview with 88 subjects hospitalized for HF. Over-recruitment was performed in a sample known to have high attrition rates. Eight subjects withdrew, and 10 subjects were lost from the study because of death before the end of the 3-month follow-up period. A *t* test was run to compare the 2 groups of patients (those who died within 3 months of discharge and those who survived) on the following measures: age, NYHA class, ejection fraction, comorbidities, educational level, and initial quality of life scores. There were no significant differences on any of the measures between the 2 groups. The final sample consisted of 37 control and 33 treatment subjects. The sample characteristics are shown in Table I.

Table II lists demographic characteristics, presence of visiting nurse follow-up (Visiting Nurse Association), and medication use in the sample. Chi-square analysis demonstrated no significant differences between the treatment and control group on any of the characteristics listed in Table II. The sample size provided adequate power for all outcome variables.

INSTRUMENTS

Heart failure readmission rates

The outcome variable of HF readmission rates was measured by counting the total number of admissions for HF in each group during the 3-month study interval. Each admission counted as 1 number, regardless of the number of days admitted.

Quality of life

The variable of quality of life was measured with the Minnesota Living with Heart Failure (MLHF) questionnaire.[47] The MLHF is a disease-specific 21-item measure of health-related quality of life. Patients with HF rate their perceptions about how much HF impacts their

TABLE I

Characteristics of the sample

	Treatment group (n = 33)		Control group (n = 37)	
	Mean	SD	Mean	SD
Age	75.70	12.25	76.84	10.48
NYHA	3.00	0.62	3.00	0.57
EF	41.45	18	38.75	19.5
No. of comorbidities	3.67	2	3.96	2
Education (y)	11	3.71	11	2.24

ATHA, New York Heart Association; EF, ejection fraction.

TABLE II

Sample demographic, visiting nurse, and medication use characteristics

	Treatment group (n = 33)		Control group (n = 37)	
	Frequency	%	Frequency	%
Marital status				
Single	6	8.6	7	10
Married	12	17.1	13	18.6
Widowed	13	18.6	14	20
Divorced/separated	2	2.9	3	4.3
Race				
White	31	93.9	33	89.2
Black	2	6.1	4	10.8
Gender				
Female	16	48.5	21	56.8
Male	17	51.5	16	43.2
Medications				
Beta blockers				
Yes	18	54.5	16	43.2
No	15	45.5	21	56.8
ACE inhibitors				
Yes	19	57.6	24	64.9
No	14	42.4	13	35.1
Lasix				
Yes	28	84.8	31	83.8
No	5	15.2	6	16.2
Digoxin				
Yes	15	45.5	14	37.8
No	18	54.5	23	62.2
VNA services				
Yes	17	51.5	17	45.9
No	16	48.5	20	54.1

ACE, Angiotensin-converting enzyme; VNA, Visiting Nurse Association.

socioeconomic, psychologic, and physical aspects of daily life, from 0 (not at all) to 5 (very much). Scores on the total instrument range from 0 to 105, with higher scores reflective of worse perceived quality life. Construct validity was demonstrated by significant correlations of MLHF scores with NYHA functional classifications in 83 subjects with HF caused by left ventricular dysfunction ($r = .80$, $P < .01$).[48] Significant correlations were also noted between the MLHF and a single-item measure that rated overall how much HF prevented them from living as they wanted in the past month ($r = .80$, $P < .01$). Internal consistency reliability on the instrument is high, with Cronbach's alpha of 0.94 reported for the total scale.[49] The Cronbach's alpha for the total scale in this study was 0.87.

Benefits and barriers

The instruments used to measure the benefits and barriers of taking HF medications, following a sodium-restricted diet, and self-monitoring for signs of fluid overload are the Health Belief Scales developed by Bennett and colleagues (personal communication, Susan J. Bennett, RN, DNS, FAAN, 2003).[49,50] The 3 scales are based on the HBM and consist of the Beliefs About Diet Compliance Scale (BDCS), Beliefs About Medication Compliance Scale (BMCS), and Beliefs About Self-Monitoring Compliance Scale (BSMCS). Each scale consists of a benefit and barrier subscale that describes potential benefits or barriers to taking HF medications, following a sodium-restricted diet, or self-monitoring for signs of fluid overload. The BDCS and BMCS each contain 12 items and the BSMCS contains 18 items. The total number of items is 42.

A Likert-type scale is scored from 1 to 5, with 1 corresponding to "strongly disagree" and 5 corresponding to "strongly agree," with the benefit or barrier item presented. The benefit and barrier subscale scores for each of the 3 scales are summed, with a range determined by the number of benefit and barrier items in the subscale. The BDCS has 5 benefit and 7 barrier items. The barrier scores range from 7 to 35, and the benefit scores range from 5 to 25. The BMCS contains 6 benefit and 6 barrier items, so the scores for both subscales range from 6 to 30. The BSMCS contains 12 barrier questions and 6 benefit questions and scores on benefit questions range from 6 to 30, and barrier scores range from 12 to 60.

Internal consistencies of the BDCS and BMCS subscales were psychometrically evaluated in a convenience sample of 101 clients with HF. Internal consistencies of these 2 subscales were found to be 0.87 for benefits of medications, 0.91 for barriers to medications, 0.84 for benefits of diet, and 0.69 for barriers of diet.[50] Content validity of the tool was found when evaluated by 2 HF experts, with 81% agreement on the content.

In this study, internal consistencies of the subscales were 0.80 for benefits of medications, 0.72 for barriers of medications, 0.85 for benefits of diet, 0.62 for barriers of diet, 0.89 for benefits of self-monitoring, and 0.83 for barriers of self-monitoring. Bennett and colleagues[50] suggest that the barriers to diet subscale score may be slightly less the others because of the heterogeneous nature of that subscale. A confirmatory factor analysis was performed on the BDCS and the BMCS in a sample of 234 persons with HF.[51] A 2-factor solution (benefits and barriers) resulted from the analysis (n = 196) of the BMCS items, accounting for 41% of the variance. In the analysis of the BDCS, a similar 2-factor solution (benefits and barriers) emerged that represented 50% of the variance. All but 1 item loaded more than 0.40.

Demographic data were collected with a tool developed by the researchers and obtained during a preliminary chart review and interview while the subject was hospitalized. Additional data were collected on medication changes during each intervention session.

PROCEDURE

Approvals were received from the institutional review board at the community hospital where the study was conducted. Two baccalaureate-prepared research nurses enrolled participants and completed the study intervention as outlined in a detailed protocol. Weekly meetings were held between the coinvestigators and the research nurses to review the protocol, answer any questions, and update the status of data collection. Periodic practice with delivering the intervention according to the protocol was performed during these meetings to prevent treatment drift.

After stabilization of HF, hospitalized subjects were invited to participate in the study, and written informed consent was obtained. After consent, subjects were randomly assigned to groups using the sealed envelope technique.[52] An interview was conducted with subjects by the research nurse during initial hospitalization to obtain relevant demographic data and complete the MLHF tool. Subjects in the treatment group were interviewed using the Health Belief Scales to determine areas in which teaching was needed. Additional demographic and medication data were obtained from the medical record and computerized hospital databases.

In a follow-up visit, 7 to 10 days after hospital discharge, the research nurse who enrolled the subject visited the subject in his or her home and again completed The Health Belief Scales. Medication lists were reviewed, and any medication changes were noted. An analysis of medications was performed to monitor changes in medications that might impact readmission rates. Prior research suggests that readmission may occur because of difficulty adjusting to medication changes.[8] The final follow-up visit took place 1 month after discharge in the subject's home, and the same research nurse again visited the subject. Quality of life scores were determined at the final interview, and medications were reviewed for any changes. A telephone call was made to the control subjects by a blinded data collector at 1 month to determine quality of life scores using the MLHF. The outcome variable of HF readmission rates was obtained through both the hospital computerized database and a telephone call by a blinded data collector to all subjects at 3 months to assess whether they had been readmitted to a hospital other than the initial hospital.

INTERVENTION

Treatment subjects

Subjects in the treatment group received a tailored message intervention by the same research nurse during hospitalization and 1 week and 1 month after hospital discharge. All subjects assigned to the treatment group received the intervention. The intervention was based on the perceived benefits and barriers to self-care of HF that were identified by persons with HF. An evaluation of health beliefs was performed using the Health Belief Scales. Questions on the Health Belief Scales are divided into benefit and barrier questions based on the HBM definitions of those terms. At each time period, subjects in the treatment group were administered all 3 scales of the Health Belief Scales. Items on the scales were scored, and if the person with HF scored 4 or above on a benefit question or below 3 on a barrier question, then a tailored message was not given. It is presumed that the person with HF already understands the barriers or benefits identified in that question. Subjects who scored outside these parameters received a message tailored to the benefit or barrier item identified in the statement (messages based on those developed by Susan J. Bennett).[49] The messages used in this study were a shortened version of those developed by Susan J. Bennett, but they included the same content. The total time for administration of the tailored message intervention averaged 15 minutes per participant. Written copies of the messages were not given to the participants. Examples of tailored messages used in this study are presented in Table III.

Control subjects

Subjects in the control group received usual care, which included discharge teaching by a staff nurse on the unit and written educational sheets describing the uses, side effects, and frequency of any ordered medications. In addition, approximately one half of the subjects also received referrals to local visiting nurse agencies. After enrollment, the control subjects were contacted at 1 month by a blinded data collector to evaluate quality of life and at 3 months to evaluate readmission rates.

ANALYSIS

Data were entered into the Statistical Package for Social Sciences 10.0 (SPSS Inc, Chicago, IL), and descriptive statistics were computed on all study variables and examined for the presence of random or systematic missing data, significant skewness, and outliers. Appropriate reli-

TABLE III
Sample tailored messages

Diet	
Benefit question: Salty food is not good for me.	Barrier question: Food does not taste good on a low-salt diet.
Message: Salt is not good for you because salt causes your body to hold more water. When your body holds more water then your heart has to work harder to pump blood through your body.	Message: After you have followed the low-salt diet a while, you will get used to the taste of the foods. Foods can still be flavored with other spices and also salt substitutes. You can see a dietitian or refer to cookbooks on low-salt cooking.

Medications	
Benefit question: If I take my water pills, I will lower my chance of being hospitalized.	Barrier question: Taking water pills makes it hard to go away from home.
Message: Taking your pills at the time and in the amount ordered by your doctor will help keep your body from holding extra fluid. Getting rid of this extra fluid will prevent swelling in your body and may make you feel better.	Try to take your pills earlier in the day when you are going out so that they will work before you leave the house. Also, when you go out be sure to find the bathroom wherever you go.

Reprinted with permission of the author, Dr. Susan J. Bennett.

ability and validity measures were performed on measurement instruments. Because the outcome variable of HF readmission rates was skewed, the nonparametric Kruskall-Wallis statistic was computed to determine differences in HF readmission rates between the treatment and control groups. The benefits, barriers, and quality of life data were not skewed. Repeated-measures analysis of variance (ANOVA) was performed to compare the quality of life scores at baseline and 1 month between the treatment and control groups. A repeated-measures ANOVA was run on the benefits and barriers scores at 3 time points to determine whether there were significant differences in benefit and barrier beliefs over time. Subjects who withdrew or died before the 3-month follow-up point were excluded from the analyses.

RESULTS
Readmission rates

A Kruskall-Wallis test was run to answer research question 1. HF readmission rate was not significantly related to group assignment in this study ($P = .22$). As seen in Table IV, 12 subjects in the control group were rehospitalized 1 or more times, whereas 6 subjects in the treatment group were rehospitalized 1 or more times.

TABLE IV
Heart failure readmission rates by group

Number of HF readmissions	Treatment (n = 33) No. (%)	Control (n = 37) No. (%)	Total HF readmissions No. (%)
0	27 (82)	25 (68)	52 (74)
1	3 (9)	9 (24)	12 (17)
2	3 (9)	2 (5)	5 (7)
3	0 (0)	1 (3)	1 (1)

Statistical test = Kruskall-Wallis. P = .22. HF, Heart failure.

TABLE V
Changes in benefits and barrier scores over time

	Baseline M (SD)	1 wk M (SD)	1 mo M (SD)	df	F	P
Benefits of medications	21.2 (3.6)	22 (2.1)	22.2 (3.7)	2	1.381	.259
Barriers of medications	15.5 (4.1)	15.1 (3.8)	13.3 (3.2)	2	12.627	.000*
Benefits of diet	25.2 (5)	28.2 (2.7)	29.7 (3.8)	2	11.890	.000*
Barriers of diet	13.6 (3.6)	11.8 (2.3)	10.4 (3.5)	2	10.145	.001*
Benefits of self-monitoring	19.8 (5.6)	22 (3.9)	23.5 (3.2)	2	10.356	.000*
Barriers of self-monitoring	27.9 (9.3)	23.8 (4.9)	22.4 (5.2)	2	8.897	.002*

*Greenhouse-Geisser epsilon correction factor used.

Quality of life

A repeated-measures ANOVA comparing quality of life by group assignment over time was performed to answer research question 2. The assumption of equality of covariance matrices was met. Because Mauchly's test of sphericity was not significant, univariate results are reported.[53] For within-subjects effects, there were significant differences in quality-of-life measures at the 2 time points (F = 35.44, P = .000), with both groups reporting improved quality of life at 1 month as expected with a group recruited during hospitalization. The mean quality of life score was 55.5 at baseline and 41.6 at 1 month. The assumption of homo-geneity of variance for between-subjects factors was met.[53] There were no significant differences between the group receiving the tailored message intervention and the control group in reported quality of life (F = 1.051, P = .309). The control group had a mean score of 50.9, and the treatment group had a mean score of 46.2. There was no significant interaction between quality of life and group assigned (F = .317, P = .575).

Benefits and barriers

To answer research question 3 (Table V), a within-subjects repeated-measures ANOVA was run to compare benefit and barrier scores of diet, medications, and self-monitoring at baseline, 1 week, and 1 month in the group receiving the tailored message intervention (n = 33).

In Table V, the mean scores for benefits of medications, diet, and self-monitoring were lowest at the baseline period and highest at 1 month follow-up. Conversely, the barriers of diet, medications, and self-monitoring were noted to be highest at baseline and lowest at 1 month. Because Mauchly's test of sphericity was significant for all but the benefits of medications data, univariate tests with the Green house-Geisser epsilon correction factor are reported.[53] The benefits of medications scores did not change significantly during the study ($P = .259$). Barriers of medications scores decreased from baseline to the 1-week point ($P = .000$) and significantly decreased from baseline to the 1-month point ($P = .000$). Benefits of diet significantly increased from baseline to 1 week ($P = .000$) and from baseline to 1 month ($P = .000$). The barriers of diet significantly decreased from baseline to 1 week ($P = 000$) and from baseline to 1 month ($P = .001$). The benefits of self-monitoring significantly improved from baseline to 1 week ($P = .000$) and from baseline to 1 month ($P = .000$). Barriers of self-monitoring decreased significantly from baseline to 1 week ($P = .002$), with further decreases at 1 month. All changes occurred in the expected theoretic directions.

DISCUSSION

Although overall HF readmission rates between the treatment and control groups did not differ significantly, fewer individuals in the treatment group were readmitted during the 3-month follow-up period (6 vs 12). The 35% of subjects rehospitalized in this study is comparable to rates reported in the literature of 29% to 66% for other samples with HF.[11,54,55] Previous research has demonstrated that persons with HF are frequently readmitted for the same reason as their primary admission because a period of time is required for stabilization of fluid status and adjustment to new medication doses.[8] With shorter lengths of hospital stay, elderly subjects with HF have not had the time to adjust physiologically to altered doses or additional medications. As a result, this population would benefit from more close home monitoring and routine referral for visiting nurse follow-up. In this sample, only slightly more than half of the subjects reported receiving home follow-up (Table II).

This intervention was a tailored message intervention and did not account for the medical management of persons with HF in the study. Clinical practice guidelines recommend the use of angiotensin-converting enzyme (ACE) inhibitors, digoxin, and diuretics in the management of HF and its associated symptoms.[3,56] As seen in this study, approximately half of all subjects were receiving beta-blockers and digoxin, approximately 60% were receiving ACE inhibitors (Table II), and 84% were receiving diuretics. These findings are consistent with those reported in the literature for patterns of use of medications for HF. Luzier and colleagues[57] reported digoxin use in 72%, diuretic use in 86%, and ACE inhibitor use in 67% of 314 subjects with HF. Oka and colleagues[58] reported digoxin use in 70%, ACE inhibitor use in 60%, and diuretic use in 95% of subjects with HF. Doyle et al[59] reported that 60% of subjects with HF were not receiving ACE inhibitors, even when no contraindications were noted, and Kermani et al[60] reported that 48% of 107 subjects with HF were not receiving ACE inhibitors on admission to the hospital. Sneed and colleagues[61] reported comparable rates with 77% receiving ACE inhibitors, 27% receiving beta-blockers, and 77% receiving diuretics in a study of persons with HF (n = 30) in an outpatient clinic. The evidence suggests a pattern of underuse of medications for HF that can lead to poor medical stabilization of the condition and render educational interventions ineffective in reducing rehospitalization rates. Without proper medical stabilization, educational interventions may be ineffective in reducing rehospitalization rates.

The quality of life results in this study are comparable to other studies. In this study, no difference in quality of life scores was noted between the 2 groups at baseline and 1 month. However, significant differences were noted in quality of life at the 1-month follow-up point across both groups. These results indicate that quality of life improved independently of intervention after hospital discharge in both groups. This finding is consistent with other studies that have shown quality of life scores to be lowest in persons with HF during hospitalization and to improve during the discharge period even in a group that does not receive intervention.[62,63] A reduction in symptoms and resulting improvement in functional status because of stabilization of symptoms during hospitalization may account for these changes in this population, because the MHLF is a disease-specific measure of quality of life. It is possible that persons who were lost to follow-up may have reported worse quality of life, so these results must be interpreted with caution.

Perhaps the length and dose of intervention can impact the perception of quality of life of the person with HF.[64] In this study, subjects received an intervention consisting of 3 nursing visits, which may have been insufficient to impact quality of life as measured by the MLHF. This finding is supported with previous research indicating that the dose of the intervention can impact specific outcomes of persons with HF. In a secondary analysis of data collected from 7 sites across the United States, it was found that persons with HF who received a more intensive intervention had greater improvement in quality of life scores than those who received a less-intensive intervention. Subjects receiving interventions over a longer period of time or with more components (education, exercise, and medication management) reported significantly improved quality of life.[63] For example, Oka and colleagues[58] reported significant improvements in quality of life scores in a group who received a 3-month exercise intervention (consisting of exercise 3-5 days/week), but a comparable group of control subjects showed no improvements. Perhaps the intensity of this intervention

was insufficient to demonstrate statistically significant changes in quality of life in the treatment group.

Although changes in quality of life scores in the treatment group did not reach statistical significance, the treatment group did report greater improvement in quality of life at 1 month than the control group. Prior research suggests that a 5-point change in the quality of life score is clinically significant in persons with HF.[47,59] Because the MLHF was developed as a disease-specific measure of the perception of function and impact of symptoms on function of the person with HF,[47,61] this finding may represent a reduction in symptoms and improved function for both groups. This finding supports other research suggesting that quality of life may be lowest during hospitalization and improve because of stabilization of symptoms resulting in improved function.[63] On the basis of this criterion, the subjects in both groups reported a statistically and clinically significant improvement in quality of life over time.

Perhaps the strongest finding of this study was that the benefit and barrier scores progressed in the expected theoretic directions. This tailored message intervention without written supplementation was able to create significant changes in health beliefs in a small group of persons with HF. Champion and colleagues[65] found that women who received a tailored message intervention that evaluated specific health beliefs (benefits, barriers, and self-efficacy) combined with practice of psychomotor skills needed to perform breast self-examination were more likely to perform the examination and do it correctly. Other theoretically guided tailored message interventions have been successfully used to reduce smoking behaviors, improve mammography screening behaviors, and improve unhealthy dietary behaviors.[66–69]

In each of these studies, subjects received tailored instruction with personalized written reminders based on an evaluation of benefit or barrier beliefs, self-efficacy beliefs, or stage of change. Subjects receiving tailored education in each of these studies reported reading the literature provided, demonstrating correct performance of self-care behaviors, and changing unhealthy dietary behaviors more often then those in the control situations. This suggests that belief patterns can be influenced by education and that perhaps an evaluation of beliefs should be included in any intervention in which behavior change is an outcome.

IMPLICATIONS

The results of this study demonstrate that a tailored message intervention changed the perceived benefit and perceived barrier of self-care of HF beliefs in this population. The psychoeducational focus of the intervention included facets of self-care that are traditionally part of home-based HF education but were tailored to the specific beliefs of the person with HF This reduced redundancy of the education. The messages in this study were easy to deliver, took approximately 15 minutes, and were suitable for delivery by telephone. In this era of cost consciousness, a reduction in the number of nursing visits and minimization of educational redundancy could be useful in the home care setting. This intervention requires testing in a larger sample of persons with HF to determine for whom the intervention would be most effective.

Although changes in benefits and barrier beliefs did occur in this study, the effect of changes on beliefs and actual self-care practice is an important consideration because actual self-care behavior change would be one potential positive outcome. Certainly the impact of other factors such as physicians or nurses providing education to these subjects could have influenced the findings and should be considered in future research. Future research that focuses on the effect of tailored interventions on actual changes in self-care behaviors and the dose of intervention needed to effect these changes would be beneficial.

LIMITATIONS

There were 3 limitations to this study. The first limitation is the lack of measurement of the actual self-care behaviors of this sample. Although beliefs were measured and did change, actual self-care behaviors, including following a low-sodium diet, daily weighing, and taking medication, were not measured. Future study should include these variables to determine whether a change in beliefs translates to actual behavior change. Second, a number of participants were lost to follow-up because of death or withdrawal and therefore were not included in the analysis. The final outcome measure was evaluated 3 months after the intervention was delivered. Some of the subjects lost to follow-up may have had worse outcomes, but these were not evaluated because of loss to follow-up. Finally, health beliefs were not measured in both the treatment and control subjects because of the nature of the intervention. Because the intervention was based on an evaluation of the health beliefs determined by the Health Belief Scales, the authors thought that administering the scales at 3 time points to control subjects was similar to the intervention given to the treatment subjects. Future study should include administration of the scales to both groups for a more accurate comparison of health belief changes over time.

The authors thank Drs. Diane Carroll, Susan Chase, and Ellen Mahoney for thoughtful review of an earlier version of this article. The authors also thank Stacey Just, BSN, RN, and Denise Tailby, BSN, RN, for assistance with data collection. Finally, the authors thank the staff of the PCU and TCU at St Luke's Hospital for assistance with identifying appropriate subjects for the study.

REFERENCES

1. American Heart Association. 2002 Heart and Stroke Statistical Update. Dallas: American Heart Association; 2001.
2. Brashers VL. Alterations of cardiovascular function. In: McCance KL, Heuther SE, eds. Pathophysiology, 4th edition. St Louis: Mosby; 2002. p. 980-1047.

3. Hunt SA, Baker DW, Chin MH, Cinquegrani MP, Ganiats TG, Goldstein S, et al. ACC/AHA guidelines for the evaluation and management of chronic heart failure in the adult: a report by the American College of Cardiology/American Heart Association Task Force on practice guidelines. American College of Cardiology website. Available at: http://www.acc.org/clinical/ guidelines/failure/hf_index.htm. Accessed February 2. 2003.

4. Barella P, Monica ED. Managing congestive heart failure at home. AACN Clin Issues 1998;9:377-88.

5. Carlson B, Riegel B, Moser DK. Self-care abilities of patients with heart failure. Heart Lung 2001;30:351-9.

6. Jaarsma T, Abu Saad H, Halfens R, Dracup K. Maintaining the balance: nursing care of patients with chronic heart failure. Int J Nurs Stud 1997;34:213-21.

7. Happ MB, Naylor MD, Roe-Prior M. Factors contributing to rehospitalization of elderly patients with heart failure. J Cardiovasc Nurs 1997;11:74-84.

8. Anderson MA, Hanson KS, DeVilder NW. Unplanned hospital readmissions: a home care perspective. Nurs Res 1999;48: 299-307.

9. Krumholz HM, Parent E, Tu U, Vaccarino V, Wang Y, Radford MI, et al. Readmission after hospitalization for congestive heart failure among Medicare beneficiaries. Arch Intern Med 1997;157:99-104.

10. Shipton S. Risk factors associated with multiple hospital readmissions. Home Care Provid 1996;1:83-5.

11. Vinson IM, Rich MW, Sperry JC, Shah AS, McNamara T. Early readmission of elderly patients with congestive heart failure. Heart Lung 1990;38:1290-5.

12. Rich MW, Beckham V, Wittenberg C, Leen C, Freedland KE, Carney RM. A multidisciplinary intervention to prevent readmission of elderly patients with heart failure. N Engl J Med 1995;333:1190-5.

13. Rich MW, Vinson JM, Sperry JC, Shah AS, Spinner LR, Chung MK, et al. Prevention of readmission of elderly patients with congestive heart failure. Intern Med 1993;8:585-90.

14. Naylor M, Brooten D, Jones R, Lavizzo-Mourey R, Mezey M, Pauly M. Comprehensive discharge planning for the hospitalized elderly. Ann Intern Med 1994;120:999-1006.

15. Roglieri JL, Futterman R, McDonough KL, Malya G, Karwath KR, Bowman D, et al. Disease management interventions to improve outcomes in congestive heart failure. Am J Manag Care 1997;3:1831-9.

16. Rauh RA, Schwaubauer NJ, Enger EL, Moran JF. A community hospital-based heart failure program: impact on length of stay, admission and readmission rates and cost. Am J Manag Care 1999;5:37-43.

17. Urden LD. Heart failure collaborative care: an integrated partnership to manage quality outcomes. Outcomes Manag Nurs Pract 1997;2:64-70.

18. Moser DK. Heart failure management: optimal health delivery programs. In: Fitzpatrick JJ, ed. Annual review of nursing research volume 18. New York: Springer Publishing Company; 2000. p. 91-126.

19. Smith LE, Fabri SA, Pai R, Ferry D, Heywood T. Symptomatic improvement and reduced hospitalization for patients attending a cardiomyopathy clinic. Clin Cardiol 1997;20:949-54.

20. Welsh C, McCaffery M. Congestive heart failure management: a continuum of care. J Nurs Care Qual 1996;10:24-32.

21. Elkman L, Andersson B, Ehnforst M, Mateika B, Perrson B, Fagerberg B. Feasibility of a nurse-monitored, outpatient care programme for elderly patients with moderate-to-severe, chronic heart failure. Eur Heart J 1998;19:1254-60.

22. Shah NB, Der E, Ruggeiro C, Heidenreich PA, Massie BM. Prevention of hospitalizations for heart failure with an interactive home monitoring program. Am Heart J 1998;135:173-8.

23. Riegel B, Carlson B, Kopp Z, LePetri B, Glaser D, Unger A. Effect of a standardized nurse case-management telephone intervention on resource use in patients with chronic heart failure. Arch Intern Med 2002;162:705-12.

24. Weinberger M, Oddone EZ, Henderson WG. Does increased access to primary care reduce hospital readmissions? N Engl J Med 1996;334:1441-7.

25. West JA, Miller NH, Parker KM, Senneca D, Ghandour G, Clark M, et al. A comprehensive management system for heart failure improves clinical outcomes and reduces medical resource utilization. Am J Cardiol 1997;79:58-63.

26. Brooten D, Kumar S, Brown L, Butts P, Finkler S, Bakewell-Sachs S, et al. A randomized clinical trial of early hospital discharge and home follow-up of very low birthweight infants. N Engl J Med 1986;315:834-9.

27. Naylor MD, Brooten D, Campbell R, Jacobsen BS, Mezey MS, Pauly MV, et al. Comprehensive discharge planning and home follow-up of hospitalized elders: a randomized clinical trial. JAMA 1999:281 613-20.

28. Naylor MD, McCauley KM. The effects of a discharge planning and home follow-up intervention on elders hospitalized with common medical and surgical cardiac conditions. J Cardiovasc Nurs 1999:14:44-54.

29. Naylor MD. Transitional care of older adults. In: Fitzpatrick JJ, ed. Annual review of nursing research volume 20. New York: Springer Publishing Company; 2002. p. 127-47.

30. Brooten D, Youngblut JM, Deatrick J, Naylor M, York R. Patient problems, advanced practice nurse (APN) interventions, time and contacts among five patient groups. J Nurs Scholarsh 2003:35:73-9.

31. Agency for Health Care Policy and Research. Heart failure: evaluation and care of patients with left-ventricular systolic dysfunction (AHCPR Publication no. 94-0612). Rockville (MD): US Department of Health and Human Services; 1994.

32. Dunbar SB, Jacobsen LH, Deaton C. Heart failure: strategies to enhance patient self-management. AACN Clin Issues 1998; 9:244-56.

33. Murray PJ. Rehabilitation information and health beliefs of post-coronary patients: do we meet their information needs? J Adv Nurs 1989;14:686-93.

34. Richardson HM. The perceptions of Canadian young adults with asthma of their health teaching/learning needs. J Adv Nurs 1991;16:447-54.

35. Turton J. Importance of information following myocardial infarction: a study of the self-perceived learning needs of patients and their spouse/partner compared with perceptions of nursing staff. J Adv Nurs 1998:27:770-8.

36. Wehby D, Brenner PS. Perceived learning needs of patients with heart failure. Heart Lung 1999;28:31-40.

37. Falvo DR. Education evaluation: what are the outcomes? Adv Ren Replace Ther 1995;2:227-33.

38. Lee NC, Wasson DR, Anderson MA, Stone S, Gittings JA. A survey of patient education post-discharge. J Nurs Care Qual 1998: 13:63-70.

39. Joint Commission on Accreditation of Healthcare Organizations. JCAHO accreditation manual for hospitals. Oakbrook Terrace (IL): JCAHO; 1997.

40. Becker MH. The Health Belief Model and sick role behavior. In: Becker MH, ed. The Health Belief Model: personal health behavior. Thorofare (NJ): Charles Slack; 1974. p. 82-93.

41. Maiman LA, Becker MH. The Health Belief Model: origins and correlates in psychological theory. In: Becker MH, ed. The Health Belief Model: personal health behavior. Thorofare (NJ): Charles Slack; 1974. p. 9-26.

42. Leventhal H, Cameron L. Behavioral theories and the problem of compliance. Patient Educ Couns 1987;10:117-38.

43. Sheeran P, Abraham C. The Health Belief Model. In: Connor M, Norman P, eds. Predicting health behavior: research and practice with social cognition models. Buckingham: Open University Press; 1996. p. 23-61.

44. Kasl SV. The Health Belief Model and behavior related to chronic illness. In: Becker MH, ed. The Health Belief Model: personal health behavior. Thorofare (NJ): Charles Slack; 1974. p. 106-27.

45. Rosenstock IM. Historical origins of the Health Belief Model. In: Becker MH, ed. The Health Belief Model and personal health behavior. Thorofare (NJ): Charles Slack; 1974. p. 1-9.

46. Bornstein M, Bornstein H, Cohen J. Power and precision 1.00 (computer software). Bethesda (MD): National Institute of Mental Health; 1997.

47. Rector TS, Kubo SH, Cohn JN. Patient self-assessment of their congestive heart failure part 2: content, reliability and validity of a new measure the Minnesota Living with Heart Failure Questionnaire. Heart Fail 1987;3:198-209.

48. Rector TS. Cohn JN. Assessment of patient outcome with the Minnesota Living with Heart

Failure Questionnaire: reliability and validity during a randomized, double-blind, placebo controlled trial of pimobendan. Am Heart J 1992;124:1017-24.

49. Bennett SJ, Hays LM, Embree JL, Arnould M. Heart Messages: a tailored message intervention for improving heart failure outcomes. J Cardiovasc Nurs 2000;14:94-105.

50. Bennett SJ, Milgrom LB, Champion V, Huster GA. Beliefs about medication compliance in heart failure: an instrument development study. Heart Lung 1997;26:273-9.

51. Bennett SJ, Perkins SM, Forthofer MA, Brater DC, Murray MD. Reliability and validity of the compliance belief scales among patients with heart failure. Heart Lung 2001;30:177-85.

52. Jaarsma T, Halfens H, Senten M, AbuSaad HH, Dracup K. Developing a supportive-educative program for patients with advanced heart failure within Orem's general theory of nursing. Nurs Sci Q 1998;11:79-85.

53. Munro BH. Statistical methods for health care research (4th edition). Philadelphia: Lippincott: 2002.

54. Rich MW, Freedland KE. Effect of DRGs on three-month readmission rates of geriatric patients with heart failure. Am J Public Health 1988;78:680-2.

55. Wolinsky FD, Smith DM, Stump TE, Overhage JM, Lubitz NM. The sequelae of hospitalization for congestive heart failure among older adults. J Am Geriatr Soc 1997;45:558-63.

56. Williams JF, Bristow MR, Fowler MB, Francis GS, Garson AJ, Gersh B, et al. Guidelines for the evaluation and management of heart failure. Report of the American College of Cardiology/American Heart Association Task Force. J Am Coll Cardiol 1995;26:1376-98.

57. Luzier AB, Forrest A, Adelman M, Hawari FI, Izzo JL Jr. Impact of angiotensin-converting enzyme inhibitor underdosing on rehospitalization rates in congestive heart failure. Am J Cardiol 1998;15:465-9.

58. Oka RK, Demarco T, Haskell WL, Botvinick E, Dae MW, Bolen K, et al. Impact of a home-based walking and resistance training program on quality of life in patients with heart failure. Am J Cardiol 2000;85:365-9.

59. Doyle JC, Mottram DR, Stubbs H. Prescribing of ACE inhibitors for cardiovascular disorders in general practice. J Clin Pharm Ther 1998;23:133-6.

60. Kermani M, Dua A, Gradman AH. Underutilization and clinical benefits of angiotensin-converting enzyme inhibitors with patients with asymptomatic left ventricular dysfunction. Am J Cardiol 2000;86:644-8.

61. Sneed NV, Paul S, Michel Y, VanBakel A, Hendrix G. Evaluation of 3 quality of life measurement tools in patients with chronic heart failure. Heart Lung 2001;30:332-40.

62. Reidinger MS, Dracup KA, Brecht ML, Padilla G, Sarna L, Ganz P. Quality of life in patients with heart failure: do gender differences exist? Heart Lung 2001;30:105-16.

63. Riegel B, Moser DK, Glaser D, Carlson B, Deaton C, Armola R. et al. The Minnesota Living with Heart Failure Questionnaire sensitivity to difference in responsiveness to intervention intensity in a clinical population. Nurs Res 2002;51:209-18.

64. Brooten D, Naylor MD. Nurses' effect on changing patient outcomes. J Nurs Scholarsh 1995;27:95-9.

65. Champion V, Foster IL, Menon U. Tailoring interventions for health behavior change in breast cancer screening. Cancer Pract 1997;5:283-8.

66. Campbell MK, DeVillis B, Strecher VJ, Ammerman AS, DeVillis RF, Sandler RS. Improving dietary behavior: the effectiveness of tailored messages in primary care settings. Am J Public Health 1994;84:783-7.

67. Perry CF, Bauer KD. Effect of printed tailored messaging on cancer risk behavior. Top Clin Nurs 2001:16:42-52.

68. Skinner CS, Strecher VJ, Hospers H. Physician's recommendations for mammography: do tailored messages make a difference? Am J Public Health 1994;84:43-9.

69. Lu ZYJ. Effectiveness of breast self-examination nursing interventions for Taiwanese community target groups. J Adv Nurs 2001;34:163-70.

A Phenomenological Exploration of Spirituality Among African American Women Recovering from Substance Abuse

VIOLET L. WRIGHT

Spirituality among African American women recovering from substance abuse is a recovery phenomenon: little is known about the individual's experience in this process. The ameliorating effect of spirituality covering a broad range of positive outcomes has been consistent across populations, regardless of gender, race, study design, and religious affiliation. Giorgi's phenomenological method was used to explore and describe the meaning of spirituality of 15 African American women recovering from substance abuse. The findings are described and discussed relative to the state of the science on spirituality. Implications for substance abuse and recovery practitioners are presented.
© 2003 Elsevier Inc. All rights reserved.

RECOVERY FROM SUBSTANCE abuse is a recovery phenomenon that is of importance to nursing. Reports in the literature indicate that recovery from substance abuse is a complex multidimensional process that occurs both with and without expert assistance (Prochaska, DiClemente, & Norcross, 1992). Whereas a combination of human, social, and economic costs of substance abuse have led to a plethora of research on topics such as the epidemiology of substance abuse, treatment outcomes such as client functioning, relapse phenomena, and most recently matching individual and treatment characteristics (Murphy, 1993), very little is known about recovery from substance abuse in African American women. Although studies conducted with women have increased within the last decade, those conducted may not be generalizable to African American women (Davis, 1997; Jackson, 1995; Murphy, 1993). It is estimated that women represent at least one-quarter of all who are dependent on various substances (Davis, 1997; Greenfield & Rogers, 1999). The recidivism rate for substance abusers has been reported to be at 90% 12 months after treatment, with most relapse occurring after 3 months (Substance Abuse and Mental Health Services Administration, 1996).

For many African American women recovering from substance abuse, current treatment modalities and self-help groups do not meet their needs (Hooks, 1993; Nelson-Zlupko, Dore, Kauffman, & Kaltenbach, 1996), because mainstream treatment of substance abuse has traditionally been developed and implemented by male providers for male clients (Abbott, 1994;

From Wright, V.L. (2003). A phenomenological exploration of spirituality among African American women recovering from substance abuse. Archives of Psychiatric Nursing, 17(4), 173-185. © 2003 Elsevier Inc. All rights reserved.

Reed, 1985). Unlike treatment for men, which can be individualistic oriented, women's treatment must be focused within the context of their relationship to others (Finkelstein, 1994). Research suggests that women may benefit from substance abuse programs that include a residential component, as well as gender-specific services (Dempsey & Wenner, 1996; Nelson-Zlupko, et al., 1996). Spirituality has often been noted in the health care literature to affect recovery (Ellison & Levin, 1998; McNichol, 1996; Sloan, Bagiella, & Powell, 1999).

Although there has been a proliferation of reports in the health care literature substantiating the ameliorating effects of spirituality with a broad range of positive outcomes, only a few have focused on specific spiritually derived strategies as an aid to recovery (Brome, Owens, Allen, & Vevaina, 2000; Ellison & George, 1994: Green, Fullilove & Fullilove, 1997; McMillen, Howard, Nower, & Chung, 2001). It has also become important to articulate the distinction between spirituality and religion. Although some may regard the two as indistinguishable, others believe religion has specific behavioral, social, doctrinal, and denominational characteristics, whereas spirituality is concerned with the transcendent, and addressing ultimate questions about life's meaning (Carson, 1989: McSherry & Draper, 1998; Nagai-Jackobson & Burkhardt, 1989; Reed, 1992). These differences are acknowledged. Undoubtedly, this confusion between spirituality and religion has been a huge roadblock in the understanding of what it means to be human.

An individual's unique spirituality or spiritual "style," is the way he or she seeks to find or create, use, and expand personal meaning in the context of the universe (Thibault, Ellor, and Netting, 1991). Feminist researchers and theologians have suggested that spirituality may be expressed differently by women than by men (Anderson & Hopkins, 1991; Reuther, 1992). Turner et al., (1998) concluded that ethnic minority women returned to church after beginning recovery with greater regularity than Anglo women. It is, therefore, possible that the ethnic minority churches may be meeting the needs of recovering women. The need for an Afrocentric approach in the treatment and recovery of substance abuse that would facilitate the strengthening of identity, spirituality, and community has been articulated by several researchers interested in the Afrocentric worldview (Asante, 1988; Belgrave et al., 1994; Brisbane & Womble, 1985). Spirituality is considered to be the cornerstone of activities within the African American community (Jackson, 1995; Scandrett, 1994). Most of these activities are centered around the Black Church. How spirituality might be used in recovery and healing needs to be explored and described in this population.

Since the conception of modern nursing by Nightingale, spirituality has been central to the essence of nursing. In providing holistic care, nursing now addresses spirituality. The concept that the provision for patients' spiritual needs is encompassed within the nurse's role is supported by prolific nursing writers such as Carson (1989) and nurse theorists like Watson (1988), Roy (1984), Neuman (1989), and Reed (1992). Nurses are obligated to care for the whole human being, presupposing that they understand and accept patients' spiritual experiences irrespective of their ways of expressing them. Therefore, the first step is for nurses and other health care professionals to begin their own spiritual journeys. As nurses achieve awareness of their inner selves, they can more readily address the spiritual needs of others by looking beyond the physical and more deeply within, and become aware that there is something sacred that can be witnessed and shared in the midst of life's illness and disease. A phenomenological understanding of all that spirituality may represent to African American women is relevant to the recovery process from substance abuse.

PURPOSE

A qualitative phenomenological research study was designed to explore the essential elements of the lived experience of spirituality among African American women recovering from substance abuse, and to describe the meanings made of this phenomenon by the person experiencing it.

METHODS

Philosophical Perspective

The perspectives of Frankl (1965,1984) provide the conceptual orientation for this study, whereas direction for data analyses was provided by the procedural steps of Giorgi's (1985) method. Frankl (1984) states that the meaning of life differs from man to man, from day to day, and from hour to hour. Frankl (1984) proposed that the chief dynamic behind the addictive behavior is "existential frustration" created by a vacuum of a perceived meaning in personal existence, and manifested by the symptom of boredom. The underpinnings of Frankl's work stresses individual's freedom to transcend suffering and find meaning in life regardless of his circumstances. The substance abuser often looks on his existence as meaningless and without purpose. Frankl's (1984) concept of how meaning in life differs from day to day correlates with the philosophies of Alcoholics Anonymous (AA) in their statement about staying sober "one day at a time." Frankl's (1984) work is based on empirical or phenomenological analysis, which was described as the way in which man understands himself, and how he interprets his own existence.

Methodology

Phenomenology was chosen as the methodology for this study, in that it describes the world as it is experienced before any theories being devised to explain it. The aim of phenomenology in nursing research is to describe the experience of others so that those who care for these individuals may be more empathetic and understanding of the person's experience.

Phenomenology seeks meanings from appearances and arrives at essences through intuition and reflection on conscious acts of experiences, leading to ideas, concepts, judgements, and understandings. The core processes included in the phenomenological methodology are epoche or bracketing, phenomenological reduction (intuiting), imaginative variation (analyzing), and synthesis of meanings and essences (describing). Bracketing involves refraining from judgment, abstaining or staying away from the everyday or ordinary way of seeing things. In our natural attitude we tend to hold knowledge judgmentally, we presuppose that what we perceive in nature is actually there and remains there as we perceive it. Giorgi describes this process as setting aside one's own presuppositions or knowledge about a particular phenomenon. Intuiting involves the task of describing in textural language, just what one sees, not only in terms of the external object but also the internal acts of consciousness. The reduction is strictly a methodological move to temporarily strip the world of the multitude of implicit presumptions about its existence as "real" thereby allowing aspects of the world to occur as pure phenomena for consciousness. The term imaginative variation or analyzing means "to arrive at structural descriptions of an experience, the underlying and precipitating factors that account for what is being experienced" (Moustakis, 1994), p. 98. Giorgi refers to this process as the delineation of "meaning units" and that by freely changing aspects or parts of a phenomenon or object one is able to see if the phenomenon remains identifiable or not. Characteristics that describe a phenomenon are imagined or condensed thoroughly by the researcher and those elements that clearly describe and are characteristic of the phenomenon are considered essential. Describing involves the integration of textural language into a unified statement of the essences of the experience of the phenomenon under investigation. It is describing the central characteristics of the phenomenon by using analogy, negation, and metaphor.

METHODS

Within phenomenological methodology, there are several schools of thought, and various methods for collecting and analyzing data (Ornery, 1983; Spiegelberg, 1982). The types of method are closely associated with the philosophical/theoretical perspectives. For this study, Giorgi's (1985) phenomenological method was chosen. Selecting Giorgi was based on three factors: First, for its well-defined method which was influenced by the works of Husserl (1913/1931) and Merleau-Ponty (1962), secondly, the ability to use psychological analysis of interpretation in formulating meaning units with greater clarity, and third, the researcher is able to analyze the descriptions with a special sensitivity to the perspective of his or her discipline. When analyzed from within a disciplinary framework, Giorgi defines the meaning units as the scientific essences. Thus, his method appeared particularly well suited for the exploration of phenomena, which is of concern for psychiatric-mental health and substance abuse and recovery nursing. Giorgi makes clear that it is critical to distinguish between the use of philosophical phenomenology, which is universal and foundational, and the use of the empirical phenomenological approach that seeks to disclose and elucidate the phenomena of behavior as they present themselves.

This study followed the core processes of phenomenology and the four steps outlined in Giorgi's (1985) method, which are as follows: (1) The researcher reads the entire description of the learning situation obtained from the participants to get a sense of the whole statement; (2) next, once a sense of the whole has been grasped, the researcher rereads the same description more slowly with the specific intent of discriminating "meaning units" from within a psychological perspective and with a focus on the phenomenon of interest; (3) once the "meaning units" have been delineated, the researcher then goes through all of the "meaning unit" and expresses the psychological insight contained in them more

directly. This is especially true of the meaning units more revelatory of the phenomenon under consideration: (4) finally, the researcher synthesizes the transformed meaning units.

STUDY PARTICIPANTS

The number of participants was determined by the number of persons required to permit an indepth exploration and obtain a clear understanding of the phenomenon of interest from various perspectives. This occurred with 15 participants when data saturation was achieved, with no new themes or essences emerging from the participants and the data were repeating. Participants were recruited froth a women's shelter with the help of a colleague as contact person, from church support groups within the community by the researcher who made church members aware of the study and the search for participants, and through networking, whereby each participant interviewed suggested the name of a potential new participant.

Each participant met the following criteria: over 18 years of age; identified herself as an African American woman; substance free status for at least 1 year; able to participate and engage in interviews of 1 to 2 hours in length; expressed interest in participating in the study; not currently being treated for psychotic disorders; and was able to read and write in the English language. There was no restriction as to the length of substance abuse to enter the study.

There were 15 participants who ranged from 29 to 49 years of age. With respect to marital status, the majority—eight of the participants were never married, whereas six were divorced and one currently married. The participants reported a mixed range of religious affiliation, with all of them considering themselves to be Christians. Seven participants attended religious activities more than once per week. All the participants reported an increase in their spirituality since becoming drug free. All participants identified their higher power as God or Jesus Christ.

Of the participants 12 began using substances between the ages of 5 to 12, with all having some form of structured treatment for substance abuse. A majority of the participants reported having past legal problems. With respect to abstinence eight participants reported 7-12 years of drug free status. and seven having 15-39 months of substance free status.

PHENOMENOLOGICAL RIGOR

Guba (1991) suggests that credibility, dependability, confirmability, and transferability be used to support rigor in qualitative research. Although Giorgi's (1985) phenomenological analysis does not rely on participant review or intersubjective agreement by expert judges, peer debriefing, or returning to participants to validate findings to establish qualitative rigor, some aspects of rigor drawn from Lincoln & Guba's (1985) work were applied to increase trustworthiness of the interpretation. Streubert and Carpenter (1995) states that rigor or trustworthiness in qualitative research can be achieved through the researcher's attention to and confirmation of the information discovered (p. 25). The goal of maintaining rigor is to accurately represent what those who have been studied experience.

Credibility involves activities that increase the probability that credible findings will be produced (Lincoln & Guba, 1985). One of the best ways to establish credibility is through prolonged engagement with the subject matter. For this, Giorgi (1985) considers the process of bracketing, phenomenological reduction, and concern for essences as evidence of reliability and validity. Bracketing in this study was achieved through "journaling" throughout data collection and analysis. Notes regarding beliefs, presuppositions, and past experiences with spirituality and recovery from substance abuse, as well as thoughts after interviews were recorded and discussed with senior researchers. These entries were useful in achieving bracketing and in rendering noninfluential this researcher's prior experiences and presuppositions on the

phenomenon. Dependability is met through credibility (Streubert & Carpenter, 1995). Confirmability is the way one documents the findings by leaving an audit trail. An audit trail is a recording of activities over time. which can be followed by another individual (Streubert & Carpenter, 1995, p. 26). The objective is to clearly illustrate the evidence and thought process that led to the conclusions. The use of journals also serves to establish confirmability. In this study, presenting the data from the beginning where naive meaning units were identified, to clustering, and finally to themes and the essential descriptions achieved this end. Transferability is the probability that the findings of the study have meaning to others in similar situations.

PROCEDURE AND DATA COLLECTION

The participants were contacted in three ways: (1) through a colleague who used a woman's shelter for practice experience and had contact with African American women recovering from substance abuse, (2) from community contacts with church support group members, and (3) through networking. The purpose of the study was explained and informed consent obtained. All participants were interviewed in their homes or the shelter with each interview being audiotaped and lasting from 45 to 90 minutes. Each participant was given a brief introduction regarding the researcher's interest about the phenomenon. The interviews began with the general request: "to describe your experiences, thoughts, perceptions, and feelings of how spirituality contributed to your recovery" followed by a request to "describe an occasion or event during your substance abuse when you decided to use spirituality as a part of your recovery." Neutral probes were then used to elicit fuller description and elaboration of the experience such as "how significant is spirituality in your life?" The researcher encouraged personal perspectives to expand on the descriptions. The recall of painful memories can trigger anxiety and other emotional distress. Therefore, the emotional state of each participant was evaluated throughout the interviews by stopping when the participant was upset and offering support.

Although Giorgi's (1988) phenomenological analysis does not rely on peer debriefing, to establish qualitative rigor, notes were recorded after each interview regarding the process, feelings, and experiences of the researcher elicited by the interview. In this study during each interview the researcher was genuinely interested in participant's experience and listened honestly to their descriptions. This journaling ensured bracketing or the suspension of presuppositions on the part of the researcher. She returned frequently to what she had bracketed (the researcher's knowledge of and belief in God).

FINDINGS

After each interview was transcribed, the researcher carefully listened to the audiotape to ensure accuracy in the transcription. The narrative of each experience was then analyzed according to Giorgi's (1985) phenomenological method. In this study, the researcher read the entire description of the experience and captured the sense of the whole. Each transcript was then read and reread several times in an effort to delineate meaning units as they were conveyed in the participant's words. These are the naive meanings units, and although they are not explicitly stated by the participant they are perceived by the researcher who assumes a psychological attitude towards the concrete examples. Following this approach, the researcher identified 1669 naive meaning units in the transcribed interviews. These naive meaning units were then transformed through the process of reflection and intuitive variation into 631 formulated meaning units or constituents of the essence of spirituality for these recovering women. These essences or themes and supporting theme clusters were then formulated and later discussed in the findings. Five major themes were formulated from the narratives (Table 1). Each of these themes has supporting themes that have been extrapolated from the narratives. A typology of the themes and supporting themes were created. These themes and supporting theme clusters are not exclusive or isolated experiences but represent aspects of the participants' experiences, which sometimes are interwoven or overlap. Two examples of the themes and supporting themes are described in Table 2 to provide the reader with information about activities during the process of formulating naive-meaning units to main themes which emerged as the essence or meaning structure. Each of the themes is presented with supporting verbatims to substantiate the researcher's process in identification of themes and for the reader to grasp a full understanding of the participant's experience.

TABLE 1. Major Meaning Units
Major Themes From the Participants' Narratives

1. The absence of spirituality was experienced as abandonment when there was no personal and intimate relationship with God.

2. Spirituality was experienced as surrendering when there was a spiritual awakening.

3. The women recovering from substance abuse experienced spirituality as reconnecting when there was recognition, a realignment, and engagement with God, self, and community.

4. Spirituality was experienced as transformation when the women were able to transcend substance abuse and other difficulties and focus on restoration and growth towards new horizons.

5. Spirituality was experienced as maturation when there was attainment of newness in life.

TABLE 2. Typology of Major Themes, Naive Units, and Participant's Description

Themes	Meaning Units (MU)	Participant's Description
Example 1: The women recovering from substance experienced the absence of spirituality as abandonment when there was no personal and intimate relationship with God.	MU:1.1. The absence of spirituality was experienced as abandonment when participants recalled feeling as if something was missing from their lives, of being far from God, being in the dark, and being in bondage.	This participant experienced the absence of spirituality as abandonment by stating: "There was something missing before and I didn't know what it was. It was as if I was searching for something. And I had to go through all the hard times to find it. He shown me the light because I was in the dark."
	MU:1.2. The absence of spirituality was experienced as abandonment when the women related feeling alone and saw separation from God and others due to death or other circumstances as contributing factors.	This participant spoke of abandoning her family: "So at that Christmas dinner all my family ganged up on me and confronted me about my drug use... So I left the dinner. I didn't go to any more family gatherings for about 10 years. I abandoned my family... Even though I was clean, I didn't feel happy. I think after I stopped using, this was the loneliest period of my life. I felt alone. Like I had no one in the world."
The women recovering from substance abuse experienced spirituality as surrendering when there was a spiritual awakening.	MU:2.1. The women reported turning their lives and will over to God, letting go, relinquishing control, and putting the past behind as surrendering.	This woman stated: ". . . I had to learn how to admit that I really don't have all the answers... I surrendered my know-it-all-ism."
	MU:2.2. The women identified struggling, powerlessness, and a total dependency on God as surrendering.	This woman stated: "When I hit 18 months clean I was struggling and I was crying out to everybody. I was showing up for Bible study, I was showing up for church... I was doing all that I could do, but it wasn't enough. I still didn't have what it took on the inside... I had a dependency. I had been praying to the Lord for dependency. I said Lord I want to be totally dependent on you. So God allowed everything that I had depended on to be gone."

THE ABSENCE OF SPIRITUALITY WAS EXPERIENCED AS ABANDONMENT WHEN THERE WAS NO PERSONAL AND INTIMATE RELATIONSHIP WITH GOD

The absence of spirituality was experienced as abandonment among recovering African American women. Abandonment was alluded to in all of the narratives; however, the nature of the abandonment varied among the women in this study. The absence of spirituality was experienced as abandonment when participants reported feeling as if something was missing from their lives, of being far from God, and being in the dark. Spirituality was viewed negatively when there was the felt absence of a relationship with God. For these women abandonment was experienced as a lack of intimacy with God, which led to deterioration in fellowship and deepened into darkness. Although they lacked intimacy, they reported that after no longer using substances, realizing that their survival was a result of the unconditional abiding presence of God and that they were the ones who had abandoned God. One participant described her experience of abandonment as follows:

> . . . Although I was brought up to believe in God. at some point I still feel God failed me and I can't exactly tell where. I don't know if it was after l got married and ended up in an abusive relationship. . .For a while I had abandoned God and things in my life were going swell. But what I realize is that He hadn't abandoned me. He was just carrying this fool through so she can realize that someone was still there for her and you don't have to carry the world on your shoulders. . .

In addition, the absence of spirituality was also experienced as abandonment when ingrained knowledge of God was overshadowed by substance use. Renewed knowledge, however, resulted in God's illumination within the soul once the substance was removed and was described by one participant as follows:

> When 1 used substances, I couldn't see; I was blind. When I began not using substances, I could see God. I began to see Him.

SURRENDERING WHEN THERE WAS A SPIRITUAL AWAKENING

The lived experience of a spiritual journey begins with surrendering to God or Higher Power and can, therefore, be understood as movement towards spiritual recovery. All of the women in this study identified their belief in God and their Higher Power as referring to God or Jesus Christ. Surrendering allowed them to deal with the pain of their addiction and to hand over their life and addiction to a power greater than themselves. For these women, a spiritual awakening occurred in different ways. Some were able to recall a significant turning point or event in their recovery. One woman stated:

> I can remember very clearly the night my son got killed. He asked me to get some help. I was in the kitchen cooking . . . and he dropped to his knees and grabbed me and ask me to get some help because he didn't want to see me dead like that. Three hours later the police knocked on my door and said my son is dead. . . . Maybe he was right. That was a real spiritual awakening right there. An omen. I was like why? God took him for me to see, to get myself together. . .

One of the most genuine dimensions of surrendering for the women occurred when there was sincere repentance, purging the self, and confession. All of them spoke of the decision to turn from selfish desires and seek a higher power. The inward conviction expressed itself in outward actions. And was described by this participant as follows:

> This you have to clean up. Get rid of your old baggage. Cleaning it up. Tell on yourself. That is telling on yourself and telling God. Even though He knows, He has to know that you know what is wrong and right for you: confession. So once you told Him ok, God, I know these things are wrong with me. . . the lies, the fear. the cheating, the dishonesty. . .

THE WOMEN RECOVERING FROM SUBSTANCE ABUSE EXPERIENCED SPIRITUALITY AS RECONNECTING WHEN THERE WAS RECOGNITION, A REALIGNMENT, AND ENGAGEMENT WITH GOD, SELF, AND COMMUNITY

Participants reported their experience of reconnecting by bringing themselves to God, family, and community honestly and completely; by seeking God's guidance, and being willing to continue to face the truth of who they are, regardless of how threatening or unpleasant their perceptions may be. The spiritual journey for these women was reported to include reconnecting with the community, mainly, through AA, NA, and churches. The most significant reconnecting, however, was with their families. However, they reported that the power of faith communities—the church—provided lasting steadiness and strength for their recovery. All of the women spoke of a nuclear family. A return to the family fold was therefore perceived as reconnecting and a return to their spiritual walk or to normalcy. They were able to begin a new and different kind of learning, a learning that involved openness, honesty, patience, obedience, acceptance, forgiveness, and awareness of sense of self. This woman reported how cut off she was from her family and when reconnection occurred how she became an important part of the family again:

> Me and my husband got back together too. . . He had written me off . . . I could spend time with my family. . . I am sharing with my family and because I dropped all that negative stuff, they are able to hear me now. They are able to connect with what I am feeling.

For some of the women reconnecting was a liberation whereby dormant feelings were able to emerge, as this participant stated:

> I went to rehab and I cried more in those 28 day than I did in my 28 years of life. I was getting honest with myself for the first time. I was

brought up in a don't touch, don't talk. don't feel family. So to be able to get in touch with my feelings was something new.

Spiritual reconnection for some of the women was very difficult, but it allowed them to apologize and to be able to move on in their recovery. This participant stated:

> I made apology to my mom. I made amends to my children. I sat down and told them I really. really didn't mean to hurt you. That is who I was then. I was an addict: I can't take none of the years back. . .

SPIRITUALITY WAS EXPERIENCED AS TRANSFORMATION WHEN PARTICIPANTS WERE ABLE TO TRANSCEND SUBSTANCE USE AND OTHER DIFFICULTIES AND FOCUS ON RESTORATION AND GROWTH TOWARDS NEW HORIZONS

Transformation was experienced when the women described an inward change of something going on inside their hearts. Although some women found it "hard to describe," they were able to impart that there was a communion going on within them at all times with God. Becoming more spiritual had an ameliorating effect on these women and on their recovery, in that they were able to transcend their substance use and be spiritually transformed into God's image and become a vessel or temple and thereby receive all that He has to offer. Spiritual transformation resulted in a change in the women's thinking. The women spoke of this transformation in their thinking as a requirement for recovery. This participant stated:

> My thinking is being transformed now- in a spiritual way. He is working on me inside. Even when I mess up, 1 don't feel guilty. . . Yes, no more guilt or shame. I feel worthy now because I've let all that go: I throw all the mess in the garbage can: this was only because of my spirituality. Because of God's love. 1 am trying to transform my thinking and my heart to love and be forgiving. . .

The lived experience of spirituality for these women was experienced as a life-line in their recovery from substance abuse and as a part of their worldview—their values, customs, and beliefs. In essence spirituality became a part of their everyday life, as this participant stated:

> It is a way of life; is a way of life. . . I believe that the Creator, whom in AA 1 say Creator, but for real I mean God. Jesus Christ abides in me. So if He abides in me, then he manifest himself through me.

Another participant supported the lived experience of spirituality as part of everyday life as follows:

> When you have a belief in God. spirituality is reflected in everything that you do or say. So for me through all my years of using drugs and alcohol, I was not a spiritual person. That part was not being reflected. Today. my spirituality is being reflected in my walk and my talk. To be spiritual you have to nourish your soul, mind. and body. Your body is a temple. I was destroying mine.

Participants were spiritually transformed when they were empowered by hearing the word of God, through their church, and by reading the word of God. They described movement towards wholeness, love, and freedom as empowerment in their spiritual transformation:

> I get more and more empowered with my spirituality. 1 will pray. read the Bible all I can. . . I get deeper in touch with my God. . . My mom gave me a Bible and gave me this little booklet with verse in it. Empowering verses.

One woman described how God used her suffering to teach her and bring her closer to Him and the complex interweaving aspects of her healing process as follows:

> God has different ways of using things to get you where He wants you to be. It is a bad thing if He did that. If God did that, it's a bad thing. . . . but I have learned so much from what happened, most of all I found God.

SPIRITUALITY WAS EXPERIENCED AS MATURATION WHEN THERE WAS ATTAINMENT OF NEWNESS IN LIFE

Spiritual maturation for these women occurred when there was a constant awareness of the presence of God in their daily lives. The women reported experiencing tremendous relief in knowing God's unconditional love, in knowing that his love for them was utterly real and that prior knowledge of the worst about them could never disillusion Him about them. The women spoke of this time of crossing over from transformation as the integration of all that was learned, and claiming what has happened in their hearts. Spiritual maturation was experienced as the ability to transcend insurmountable difficulties and adversities through faith and hope. Thus healing was not only the result of faith; it also produces faith:

> . . . Now that I have come to know God . . . it doesn't matter what adversities come your way; you can still find joy. . . He will give me the strength to go on, the hope. And the faith to believe that He is there with me. That He hasn't forsaken me.

The study participants described spiritual maturation as freedom. Freedom liberated them from the past and offered an opportunity to explore problems and issues from a fresh perspective.

> It's that freedom . . . you just don't know. Freedom from the burden. Peace of mind.

For some. spiritual maturation was finding meaning and purpose in their lives.

> You may not know your purpose for tomorrow, but you know the purpose from yesterday is to get to a point of never living that way again . . . just not doing what you used to do.

And another woman stated:

> Right now the purpose is getting my kids back into my life. I haven't had them for 6 or 7 years during my recovery. . . I know this was the purpose, to be a mother to these children.

For some participants spiritual maturation was obtained by finding peace.

> Spirituality for me is being able to be in here with faith through all the storms. You know, in hard times, in crazy times. I still have peace. . . I am at peace now.

In summary, data analysis identified five themes that demonstrated the experiences of the women's spirituality in their recovery from substance abuse, which were clearly articulated in the verbatim transcripts. These themes are not exclusive or isolated experiences but represent aspects of the women's experiences, which sometimes are interwoven or overlap. This was necessary for the researcher to arrive at a plausible comprehensive understanding of the whole phenomenon.

DISCUSSION

Discussion of Findings Relevant to Literature Reviewed

The women spoke of their experience of how they lived in a state of chronic apartness, separated from God and from those who love them. Their attachment to substances usurped God, their desire for love, and their ability to love and trust. The experiences of some of the women caused them to feel that God had not only let them down but that He had set them up. As a result they put God out of their lives. Similar findings were reported (Di Lorenzo, Johnson & Bussey, 2001, and Walant, 1995) as this study, which found that separation between the self and God led to a loss of spirituality and not being able to love, trust, and nurture. It was, however, during their disconnected state that the women were able to achieve insight into their dissatisfying and destructive behavior. Loneliness and isolation are unfortunate realities in the lives of those recovering from substance abuse. The findings of this study revealed that the experience of abandonment was unique for each individual, since the interactions within one's environment are influenced by a variety of factors. As a result, the women experienced abandonment when there was loss of a significant other, or when there was overwhelming feelings of guilt due to their inability to assume roles that were critical to the sense of self and purpose in life. For the women in this study their recovery from substance abuse brought to the surface feelings such as guilt, shame, or inadequacy as a parents. These disclosures support data showing that 74% of child neglect cases involved female caregivers who abused substances (U.S. Department of Health and Human Services, 1999; Woodhouse, 1992). This study supports previous reports that childhood physical and sexual abuse as risk factors for heavy drinking among African American women can be seen as behavior to numb the pain and shame of the abuse. Early childhood trauma precipitated a downhill spiral for the women in that they felt alone and abused, and as their substance abuse escalated, they became isolated from their natural and therapeutic supports.

In this study the women's recovery from substance abuse began when they hit rock bottom, struggled and then let go by surrendering and turning their lives over to God. Surrendering contained a message that was directed toward them as they experienced themselves as utterly failing. As Farris (1994) concluded, this failure was projected onto God in such a way that the individual often believed that God sees and judges them as a failure. It was evident that their struggles and suffering had taken their toll spiritually, mentally, and physically as their narratives contained the underlying message that "all guilt will end here" by surrendering. Letting go is a fundamental principle of life. The women in this study recognized that letting go of the past was paramount to their recovery, which is in line with Chopra's (1990) conclusion that to arrive at bliss—this place of peace—one had to let go all the inbuilt words, images, emotions and activities of the mind. By letting go of the past, the women reported they were able to focus on the "now." Many of the women reported that their "know-it-all-ism" and conventional will power alone were not able to help them succeed in their recovery. An important finding in this study was that although surrendering occurred gradually for some participants. many reported having significant events that resulted in their spiritual awakening. The loss of parents. significant other, children, siblings and friends were collectively experienced by all the participants and were the catalyst for many of them surrendering and beginning their spiritual awakening.

All of the study participants recalled having previous knowledge of God some time in their lives before incorporating spirituality into their recovery from substance abuse. The central purpose for reconnecting was to know God again, but this time from a deep spiritual realm. This spiritual reconnection was experienced by going to God in prayer, reading the Bible, and worship. These activities provided them with guidance and strength in their everyday lives. However, they were able to gain extra strength in their spiritual development when they reconnected with families and groups.

The use of community was utilized by all the women in this study, as defined by Eugene (1995) and Villarosa (1994), which was a supportive community or group of people with whom one shares common beliefs and values. Although affiliations with groups such as AA and NA, which were used by some of the women, were supportive, the benefits received from their church-affiliated groups were clearly more strengthening. Some of the women spoke of "the kindred spirit" of the group, as being one in the body of Christ, which therefore made them a family. The comfort and strength received by the women were particularly important in managing the stresses of their everyday lives. Some of the women in this study spoke of "being on trial in AA and NA," some of "slowly weaning themselves away," whereas others had completely stopped using these programs as a support system. Their reasons were varied, with some reporting that these programs were just the building blocks to get them to where they were

able to find a God of their own; some felt restricted in their ability to freely give God praise for helping them to overcome their substance use; and some felt that the way the program is structured is hypocritical, in that Bill Wilson received his revelations from God for the 12 steps. which are based on the Bible. The interviewees were able to accept what Kearney (1998) spoke of as the differences of others, working on developing an identity with those of similar beliefs, and forming a community that contributed to healing. The findings of this study also supports the conclusion of Ellison and George (1994) that people's sense of existential isolation are ameliorated by knowing that they are participants in the journey of eternal significance. Through a sense of independence or autonomy, the women were able to see what Ettorre (1992) referred to as their "women-selves" as they recognized and reconnected with their past, present, and future.

Participants experienced transformation as progressive. They revealed that through fellowship with God there was daily spiritual renewal with a deepening knowledge of Him. In this study and in the literature (McMillen, Howard, Nower, and Chung, 2001; Millar and Stermac, 2000), the women spoke of their substance abuse as being a good thing, in that in the process of their substance abuse, God used the very affliction that was responsible for their demise (the old self) to effect an inward renewal and healing that lifted them above the ravishment of their disease.

All of those interviewed reported that healing for them allowed growth, which transformed their thinking. The narratives revealed that there was a spiritual transformation through the act of worshiping, whereby God communicated His presence to them, and when they learned not only to give Him thanks and make a petition, but also to worship Him by giving praise for all that He is. This is in line with Eugene's (1995) conclusion that the Black church can offer healing responses. They also reported that they were transformed by dwelling on God's word, which required devout meditation, serious study, and loyal obedience with a resulting widening grasp of the spiritual principles by which they were to grow and live. Furthermore, they disclosed that they were transformed when they were cleansed from every aspect of wrongdoing through the assurance of God's word that if they walked in obedience to the light that He gives, the blood of Christ would keep on cleansing them despite their tendency to sin. The participants' definitions of spirituality were varied, which supports previous reports of multiple definitions of spirituality in African American women (Mattis, 2000).

Maturation is an integral part of human growth and development. Spiritual maturation was the essence of recovery from substance abuse for the women in that it provided the means by which they were able to do everything. Some authors reported that African American women tend to rely on other African American women for support and that their place of worship is one of the places used in times of crisis instead of conventional counseling with therapists (Scandrett, 1994; Taylor, 2000). Most of the women in this study were single, and the church served as an integral part of their community and as a place for socialization. The literature supports the findings in this study of the women who reported that reading the Bible provided them with a sense of peace and calmness, and for some it was a source of "daily bread," which gave them strength, courage, and guidance (Green, Fullilove, & Fullilove, 1998). The theme of maturation in this study supports the philosophical perspective of Frankl (1984), which guided the study, in that substance abuse was the vehicle of the past that led to a deeper understanding of meaning and purpose in life for these women. When a sense of meaning and purpose in life was not found, these women experienced what Frankl (1984) described as an existential meaning-vacuum. The vacuum was filled with alcohol and drugs.

In summary, an analysis of interviews with 15 African American women supports the literature that recovery from substance abuse is experienced as a multifaceted process involving physical, cognitive, emotional, and psychosocial efforts. Spirituality was experienced as being similarly complex. Although the phenomenon of spirituality has received some recognition for its ameliorating properties in recovery from substance abuse, and in particular among African Americans, there are no exclusive models that address their unique needs and allow for the free expression of self and their spiritual beliefs. As the social and political turmoil continues within the substance abuse and recovery arena, and as a disenfranchised group, African American women recovering from substance abuse will continue to rely on their churches and other "faith-based programs" so that their experiences can be understood for them as a pillar within the recovery process.

LIMITATIONS

In this study, the researcher began with the assumption that all observations are value laden and made every attempt not to impose researcher bias and interpretations on the data. The study limitations, however, were the researcher having worked in psychiatry and substance abuse for many years observed a difference in the lives of African American women who had incorporated a spiritual belief in their recovery process. Most of the participants were recruited from faith-based women's shelters and church support groups; therefore, it was known that their belief was in God. This was bracketed throughout the study and participants were not directly queried about a belief in God or their religious affiliation. General open questions were used to elicit what spirituality meant to the participant.

In addition, Giorgi's (1985) method does not require peer debriefing, discussing emerging themes with study participants, and listening to their feedback to establish rigor; although these activities could help in exposing researcher bias or error. However, journaling was done to enhance self-awareness.

CONCLUSIONS AND IMPLICATIONS

The concept of spirituality is multidimensional with no clear definition. Therefore, conceptual confusion, ambiguity, and scientific skepticism have prevented adequate investigation into its potential healing effects. The lack of a clear and concise definition may in part be preventing even longer recovery for some substance abusers, who may be reluctant to incorporate this concept into their recovery because of its ambiguity. The strength of this concept as it relates to God within this inquiry has also been embraced with caution within the mental health practice and even among strong supporters of the AA model as one of the most effective ways for long-term sobriety despite its saliency. In our zeal to scientifically study, categorize, and measure spirituality, the essence of spirituality may be overlooked.

As a disenfranchised group, the significance of spirituality in the lives of African American women recovering from substance abuse is an important dimension for them to achieve meaning and purpose in their lives. Despite the efforts that have been made to address the unique needs of women in treatment and recovery programs, and in particular the needs of African American women, participants in this inquiry communicated that they experienced resistance when they expressed commitment to religious values and church participation as strategies for their ongoing recovery. Professionals working with these women must become sensitive to the culture of the African American women and integrate their cultural values into the treatment and recovery.

Because nursing espouses holistic care as a central disciplinary tenet and because of its theoretical foundation, nurses are well positioned to contribute to the understanding of the meaning of spirituality in the recovery process for African American women. Spirituality is a strength that nursing and other professionals in substance recovery can no longer afford to ignore. Nurses are called instruments of healing. Nurses, through practice strategies, can enhance the healing process of African American women recovering from substance abuse by providing supportive interventions that enhance their spiritual journey. Nursing is also concerned with human responses to stressors or illnesses. Because spirituality is increasingly being used by many people to ameliorate their pain and suffering and in their recovery, nurses need to be able to identify behaviors that indicate spirituality among these individuals. Nursing assessment and intervention for African American women using spirituality in their recovery should include a holistic approach that includes spiritual care. The power of spirituality as a component of recovery from substance abuse may be lost in a traditional analysis of recovery methods because the sense of having a relationship with or benefiting from, the guidance of a higher power or God may not be captured in standard assessments.

Any activity of life is an opportunity for nurturing the soul when performed with intention and mindfulness. Therefore, Bible study, meditating or walking in the park may provide nurture for the soul and engages one in purpose and meaning. If these are the spiritual aspects of the everyday lifeworld of the African American women recovering from substance abuse, they must be addressed by the mental health/substance abuse and recovery community in clinical practice and research if greater amelioration by spirituality is to be achieved. Only by becoming more knowledgeable about spirituality and the experiences of African American women recovering from substance abuse can nurses become a successful tool in assisting these women in their recovery.

REFERENCES

Abbott, A.A. (1994). A feminist approach to substance abuse treatment and service: Special Issue Women's health and social work, feminist perspectives. *Social Work in Health Care*, *19*, 67-83.

Anderson, S.R. & Hopkins, P. (1991). *The feminine face of God*. New York: Bantam Books.

Asante, M.K. (1988). *Afrocentricity*. Trenton, NJ: Africa World.

Belgrave, F.Z., Cherry, V., Cunningham, D., Walwyn, S., Letlaka-Rennert, K., & Phillips, F. (1994). The influence of afrocentric values. self-esteem. and black identity on drug attitudes among African American fifth graders: A preliminary study. *Journal of Black Psychology*, *20*(2), 143-156.

Brisbane, F.L., & Womble, M. (1985). Afterthoughts and recommendations. In F.L. Brisbane & M. Womble (Eds.), *Treatment of black alcoholics*. New York: Harworth.

Brome, D.R., Owens, M.D., Allen, K., & Vevaina, T. (2000). An examination of spirituality among African American women in recovery from substance abuse. *Journal of Black Psychology*, *26*(4), 470-486.

Carson, V.B. (1989). *Spiritual dimensions of nursing practice*. Philadelphia: W.B. Saunders.

Chopra, D. (1990). *Quantum healing: Exploring the frontiers of mind/body medicine*. New York: Bantam.

Davis, R.E. (1997). Trauma and Addiction Experiences of African American women. *Western Journal of Nursing Research*, *19*(4), 442-465.

Dempsey, M.D., & Wenner, A. (1996). Gender-specific treatment for chemically dependent women: A rationale for inclusion of vocational services. *Alcoholism Treatment Quarterly*, *14*, 21-30.

DiLorenzo, P., Johnson, R., & Bussey, M. (2001). The role of spirituality in the recovery process. *Child Welfare League of America*, *80*(2), 257-273.

Ellison, C.G., & George, L.K. (1994). Religious involvement, social ties, and social support in a southeastern community. *Journal for the Scientific Study of Religion*, *33*(1), 46-61.

Ellison, C.G., & Levin, J.S. (1998). The religion-health connection: Evidence, theory, and future directions. *Health Education and Behavior*, *25*(6), 700-720.

Eugene, T.M. (1995). There is a balm in Gilead: Black women and the Black church as therapeutic agents of a therapeutic community. *Women and Therapy*, *16*(2/3), 55-71.

Ettorre, E. (1992). *Women and substance abuse*. New Brunswick, NJ: Rutgers University Press.

Farris, R.F. (1994). Addiction and dualistic spirituality: Shared visions of God, self, and creation. *Journal of Ministry in Addiction & Recovery*, *1*(1), 5-31.

Finkelstein, N. (1994). Treatment issues for alcohol and drug-dependent pregnant and parenting women. *Health & Social Work*, *19*, 7-15.

Frankl, V.E. (1965, 1984). *Man's search for meaning*. New York: Simon & Schuster.

Giorgi, A. (1985). *Phenomenology and psychological research*. Pittsburgh, PA: Duquense University Press.

Green, L.L., Fullilove, M.T., & Fullilove, R.E. (1997). Stories of spiritual awakening. The nature of spirituality in recover. *Journal of Substance Abuse Treatment*, *15*(4), 325-331.

Greenfield, T.K., & Rogers, J.D. (1999). Who drinks most of the alcohol in the U. S.? The Policy Implications. *Journal of Studies on Alcohol*, *60*, 78-89.

Hooks, B. (1993). *Sisters of the yam: black woman and self-recovery*. Boston: South End.

Jackson, M.S. (1995). Afrocentric treatment of African American women and their children in a residential chemical dependency program. *Journal of Black Studies*, *26*(1), 17-30.

Kearney, M.H. (1998). Truthful self-nurturing: A grounded formal theory of women's addiction recovery. *Qualitative Health Research*, *8*(4), 495-512.

Lincoln, Y.S., & Guba, E.G. (1985). *Naturalistic Inquiry*. Beverly Hills: Sage.

Mattis, J.S. (2000). African American women's definition of spirituality and religiosity. *Journal of Black Psychology*, *26*(1), 101-122.

McMillen, C., Howard, M.O., Nower, L., & Chung, S. (2001). Positive by-products of the struggle with chemical dependency. *Journal ofSubstance Abuse Treatment*, *20*, 69-79.

McNichol, T. (1996, April 7). The new faith in medicine. *USA Today*, p. 4.

McSherry, W., & Draper, P. (1998). The debates emerging from the literature surrounding the concept of spirituality as applied to nursing. *Journal of Advanced Nursing, 27,* 683-691.

Merleau-Ponty, M. (1962). *Phenomenology of perception* (C. Smith, Trans.) London: Routledge; Kegan Paul.

Millar, G.M. & Stermac, L. (2000). Substance abuse and childhood maltreatment. Conceptualizing the recovery process. *Journal of Substance Abuse Treatment 19,* 175-182.

Moustakas, C. (1994). *Phenomenological research methods.* Thousand Oaks, CA: Sage.

Murphy, S. (1993). Coping Strategies of abstainers from alcohol up to three years post-treatment. *Image: Journal of Nursing Scholarship, 25,* 29-35.

Ngai-Jacobson, M.G.. & Burkhardt, M.A. (1989). Spirituality: cornerstone of holistic nursing practice. *Holistic Nursing Practice, 3*(3), 1-26.

Nelson-Zlupko, L., Dore, M.M., Kauffman, E., & Kaltenbach, K. (1996). Women in recovery: Their perceptions of treatment effectiveness. *Journal of Substance Abuse Treatment, 13*(1), 51-59.

Neuman, B. (1982, 1989). *The Neuman systems model: Application to nursing education and practice.* Norwalk, CT: Appleton-Century-Crofts.

Ornery, A. (1983). Phenomenology: A method for nursing research. *Advances in Nursing Science,* 5(2), 49-63.

Prochaska, J.O., DiClemente, C.C., & Norcross, J.C. (1992). In search of how people change: Application to adductive behaviors. *American Psychologist, 47,* 1102-1114.

Reed, P.G. (1985). Drug misuse and dependency in women: The meaning and implications of being considered a special population or minority group. *International Journal of Addictions, 29,* 13-62.

Reed, P.G. (1992). An emerging paradigm for the investigation of spirituality in nursing. *Research in Nursing & Health, 15,* 349-357.

Roy, C. (1984). *Introduction to nursing: An adaptation model (2nd ed).* Englewood Cliffs, NJ: Prentice-Hall.

Ruether, R.R. (1992). Motherearth, and the megamachine. In C.P. Christ & J. Plaskow (Eds.), *Womanspring rising: A feminist reader in religion.* San Francisco, CA: Harper & Row.

Scandrett, A. Jr. (1994). Religion as a support component in the health behavior of black Americans. *Journal of Religion and Health, 33,* 123-129.

Sloan, R.P., Bagiella, E., & Powell, T. (1999). Religion, spirituality, and medicine. *The Lancet, 353,* 664-67.

Spiegelberg, H. (1982). *The phenomenological movement: A historical introduction.* The Hague: Nijhoff.

Streubert, H.J., & Carpenter, D.R. (1995). *Qualitative research in nursing. Advancing the humanistic imperative.* Philadelphia, PA: Lippincott Company.

Substance Abuse and Mental Health Services Administration (1996). *Advance report number 15. In mental estimates in 1996 national household survey on drug abuse.* Washington, DC: Office of Applied Studies.

Taylor, J.Y. (2000). Sisters of the yam: African American women's healing and self-recovery from intimate male partner violence. *Issues in Mental Health Nursing, 21,* 515-531.

Thibault, J.M., Ellor, J.W., & Netting, F.E. (1991). A conceptual framework for assessing the spiritual functioning and fulfillment of older adults in long-term settings. *Journal of Religious Gerontology, 7,* 29-45.

Turner, N.H., O'Dell, K.J., Weaver, G.D., Ramirez, G.Y., & Turner, G. (1998). Community's role in the promotion of recovery from addiction and prevention of relapse among women: An exploratory study. *Ethnicity and Disease, 8,* 26-35.

U. S. Department of Health and Human Services, Administration of Children, Youth and Families (1999). *Child maltreatment 1997: Reports from the states to the National Child Abuse and Neglect Data System.* Washington DC: U. S. Government Printing Office.

Villarosa, L. (1994). The healing power of spirituality. In L.V. Villarosa (ed.), *Body & soul: The black woman's guide to physical health and emotional well-being.* New York: HarperPerennial.

Walant, K. (1995). *Creating the capacity for attachment: Treating addiction and the alienated self.* Northvale, NJ: Jason Aronson Inc.

Watson, J. (1988). *Nursing: Human science and human care.* Norwalk, CT: Appleton-Century-Crofts.

Woodhouse, L.D. (1992). Women with jagged edges: Voices from a culture of substance abuse. *Qualitative Health Research, 2*(3), 262-281.

Correlates of Recovery Among Older Adults After Major Abdominal Surgery

MARGARITE LIEB ZALON

- **Background:** Little research has examined the recovery patterns of older adults who have had major abdominal surgery.
- **Objective:** To determine whether pain, depression, and fatigue are significant factors in the return of older adults who had major abdominal surgery to functional status and self-perception of recovery in the first 3 months after discharge from the hospital.
- **Methods:** A correlational predictive study involved adults 60 years of age or older who had undergone major abdominal surgery. Data were collected during hospitalization (n = 192), then 3 to 5 days (*n* = 141), 1 month (*n* = 132), and 3 months after discharge to home (n = 126) using the Brief Pain Inventory, the Geriatric Depression Scale-Short Form, the Modified Fatigue Symptom Checklist, the Enforced Social Dependency Scale, and the Self-Perception of Recovery Scale.
- **Results:** Multiple regression analysis indicated that pain, depression, and fatigue are significantly related to patients' self-perception of recovery and functional status. Pain, depression, and fatigue explain 13.4% of the variation in functional status at 3 to 5 days, 30.8% at 1 month, and 29.1% at 3 months after discharge. These three factors also explain 5.6% of the variation in self-perception of recovery during hospitalization, 12.3% at 3 to 5 days, 33.2% at 1 month, and 16.1% at 3 months after discharge.
- **Conclusions:** Pain, depression, and fatigue are important factors to consider in the provision of care to abdominal surgery patients with a relatively uncomplicated postoperative course. Specific interventions to reduce pain, depression, and fatigue need to be evaluated for their impact on the postoperative recovery of older adults.
- **Key Words:** depression - fatigue - function recovery - pain - surgery

The leading complication of hospitalization for older patients is functional decline, which is associated with longer hospital stays, increased mortality, higher rates of institutionalization, greater need for rehabilitation and home care services, and higher costs (Inouye, Bogardus, Baker, Leo-Summers, & Cooney, 2000). Yet lengths of hospital stay for individuals 65 years of age or older decreased from 10 days in 1980 to 6 days in 2000 (National Center for Health Statistics, 2002, p. 253). Thus, nurses are responsible for facilitating patients' recovery in less time for an increasingly older population at greater risk for functional decline.

Considering nurses' greater accountability for nursing care, the nature of recovery from sur-

From Zalon, M.L. (2004). Correlates of recovery among older adults after major abdominal surgery. Nursing Research, 53(2), 99–106.

gery needs to be examined. Research has demonstrated that pain, depression, and fatigue occur after joint arthroplasty and coronary artery bypass graft (CABG), and that they occur in relation to the functional status of older adults in residential care (Gallagher, Verma, & Mossey, 2000; Liao & Ferrell, 2000; Redeker, 1993). However, few studies have specifically examined pain, depression, and fatigue in relation to the recovery of older adults after their discharge to community after major abdominal surgery. The extent of inadequate postoperative pain relief after discharge is not known. Patients may limit activities because of pain and fatigue, which then interferes with their return to their previous functional status. Depression may make the resumption of activities difficult after surgery, contributing to poorer outcomes. It is important to examine pain, depression, and fatigue together in relation to postoperative recovery because of their complex interrelations. Therefore, this study, using Levine's (1991) Conservation Model as a framework, aimed to describe the relation of pain, depression, and fatigue to recovery in older adults during the first 3 months after abdominal surgery.

Recovery from surgery is defined as improvement in functional status and the perception that one is recovering. In the context of Levine's (1991) Conservation Model, recovery is a return to wholeness that occurs by conservation of energy and restoration of integrity. Four conservation principles guide nursing practice: energy, structural integrity, personal integrity, and social integrity. Thus, when pain and depressive symptoms are decreased, energy is conserved, and when fatigue is decreased, more energy is available to the individual.

Acute pain depletes energy and generally indicates impaired structural integrity after surgery. Unrelieved pain is a persistent problem during hospitalization for surgery and after discharge (Devine et al., 1999; Moore, 1994; Redeker, 1993; Warfield & Kahn, 1995). Older patients are more likely to have persistent pain, to experience less relief from analgesics, and to

use fewer analgesics (Lay, Puntillo, Miaskowski, & Wallhagen, 1996; MacIntyre & Jarvis, 1996). Pain is a concern for patients with abdominal aortic aneurysm and older surgical patients after discharge (Galloway, Rebeyka, Saxe-Braithwaite, Bubela, & McKibbon, 1997; McDonald, 1999). Elderly women restrict their movement to deal with postoperative pain (Zalon, 1997). Decreasing movement places patients at risk for functional decline during hospitalization and after their return home.

None of the aforementioned studies examined the relation of pain to functional status in the first few months after discharge. Retirement center residents whose pain interfered with their lives rated their health as worse, were more likely to be depressed and had lower physical functioning (Gallagher et al., 2000). Older adults discharged to community after surgery may be different because of their capabilities, and may have fewer formal services available to them. However, the research suggests that older adults, because they are more likely to have unrelieved or persistent pain after surgery, are at greater risk for its interference with function and thus delaying recovery.

Depression depletes the conservation of personal integrity. The prevalence of depressive symptoms in late life is reported to be 15% (Mulsant & Ganguli, 1999). Its prevalence in older hospitalized patients ranges from 5% to 50% (Koenig, 1997; Pouget, Yersin, Wietlisbach, Bumand, & Bula, 2000). Surgery is an additional burden for older adults already at increased risk for depression, and may exacerbate the symptoms of those with some level of depression. Depression has been associated with lower functional status after colorectal cancer surgery, medical-surgical illness, and hip fracture repair (Barsevick, Pasacreta, & Orsi, 1995; Johnson, Kramer, Lin, Kowalsky, & Steiner, 2000; Mossey, Knott, & Craik, 1990), and with late mortality after CABG (Baker, Andrew, Schrader, & Knight, 2001). The relation between depression and functional status after major abdominal surgery may be similar to that associated with other surgeries because of the surgery itself, or it may be different because of the meaning attributed to the underlying illness and expectations rations about recovery. Therefore, it is important to examine depression in relation to functional status in a broader population of older surgical patients.

Fatigue is a manifestation of limited energy resources (Levine, 1991, p. 7). Postoperative fatigue has been examined in the context of a stress response model and correlated with the degree of trauma, heart rate, and deteriorating nutritional status (Christensen & Kehlet, 1993). Physiologic studies of postoperative fatigue have used small samples, have measured different variables, and generally have not examined age or functional status. A meta-analysis of postoperative fatigue intervention studies indicates that increased analgesia is effective in reducing fatigue during the immediate postoperative period after abdominal surgery (Rubin & Hotopf, 2002). However, 23 of 66 studies used fatigue measures untested for reliability and validity, and few examined functional status. Fatigue is prevalent after CABG and minimally invasive direct coronary artery bypass (Redeker, 1993; Zimmerman, Barnason, Brey, Catlin, & Nieveen, 2002). It has its most significant impact after hysterectomy during the first few months after surgery (DeCherney, Bachmann, Isaacson, & Gall, 2002). However, the cited study was a retrospective investigation of premenopausal women whose hormonal changes also may have contributed to their fatigue.

The most distressing symptoms after the discharge of patients who underwent abdominal aortic aneurysm repair are fatigue and sleep loss (Galloway et al., 1997). Abdominal surgery generally requires more time for return of bowel function, which may in turn have an impact on nutritional status and fatigue. It is not known to what extent postoperative fatigue is related to functional status or for how long. In analyzing physiologic studies, Westerblad and Allen (2002) concluded that central fatigue, referring to decreased central nervous system activation, may be more pronounced in the elderly. Liao and Ferrell (2000) found that depression, pain, number of medications, and a 3-minute walk predicted fatigue intensity among older adults in residential care, concluding that fatigue is poorly recognized and probably undertreated. Thus, older adults may be more vulnerable to the effects of postoperative fatigue on functional status. Therefore, the following research question was addressed: What is the relation of pain, depression, and fatigue to recovery, as measured by functional status and self-perception of recovery in older adults who have had major abdominal surgery?

RESEARCH DESIGN AND METHODS

Design

This study used a correlational, predictive design to measure the relation of pain, depression, and fatigue to functional status and self-perception of recovery during the first 3 months after discharge among abdominal surgery patients 60 years of age or older.

Sample

Patients 60 years of age or older who had undergone abdominal surgery were recruited from three community hospitals The criteria for inclusion in the study required that the subjects be alert and oriented, able to speak and read English, and accessible by telephone. Those who had laparoscopic surgery, neurologic dysfunction, a psychotic disorder, or surgery specifically for cancer were excluded.

Instruments

Pain Pain was measured with the Brief Pain Inventory (BPI), which was developed originally to obtain data about the prevalence and severity of pain in the general population (Daut, Cleeland, & Flanery, 1983). The BPI uses numeric scales ranging from 0 (no pain) to 10 (pain as bad as you can imagine) to measure the severity of pain (worst, least, average, right now) and pain's interference with daily life (general activity, mood, walking, work, relationships with others, sleep, and enjoyment of life). Two items related to pain relief measures were not included in the regression analysis.

The BPI has been used widely in studies involving patients with cancer. Zalon (1999) demonstrated the reliability and validity of the BPI for use with surgical patients. The Cronbach alpha reliability coefficient for the current sample ranged from .90 to .95.

Depression Depression was measured with the short form of the Geriatric Depression Scale (GDS-SF) (Sheikh & Yesavage, 1986). This 15-item yes/no checklist contains questions specifically related to geriatric depression. The GDS has been used widely with both community-dwelling elders and elderly people hospitalized for depression. The short form is correlated significantly with the long form ($r = .84$; $p \leq .001$) (Sheikh & Yesavage, 1986). The Cronbach alpha reliability coefficient for the current sample ranged from .61 to .77.

Fatigue Fatigue was measured with the Modified Fatigue Symptom Checklist (MFSC) (Yoshitake, 1971) as modified by Pugh (1993). The MFSC has 30 items (e.g., "I feel my head is heavy"; "I feel tired in my legs") measuring fatigue from a multidimensional perspective in three subscales: drowsiness, concentration, and physical symptoms measured on a 4-point Likert scale. The reliability and validity of the MFSC has been established in different clinical populations including the elderly. In the current sample, the Cronbach alpha reliability coefficient ranged from .87 to .92.

Functional Status Functional status was measured with the Enforced Social Dependency Scale (ESDS), which indicates how disease and its treatment influence patient responses by measuring the degree of assistance required to perform ordinary activities of daily living from

the patient's perspective (Benoliel, McCorkle, & Young, 1980).

The ESDS consists of 10 items in two subscales: personal and social competence. The personal competence subscale evaluates dependence on others for eating, walking, dressing, traveling, bathing, and toileting on a 6-point scale. The social competence subscale consists of activities at home, work, and recreation evaluated on a 4-point scale, and communication evaluated on a 3-point scale.

The ESDS is administered as a semistructured interview. Scores range from 10 to 51, with the higher scores indicating greater dependency. The ESDS has been used with elderly postoperative patients with cancer. The Cronbach alpha reliability coefficient for the current sample ranged from .69 to .80.

Self-Perception of Recovery after Surgery Self-perception of recovery after surgery was measured by asking participants to indicate on a 0 to 100 numeric rating scale how much they had recovered from their surgery. A single-item scale rating health in general has been used widely by the National Center for Health Statistics (Ware, Nelson, Sherbourne, & Stewart, 1992). If a participant indicated that the answer was less than 10%, clarification was sought to make sure the scale was not being confused with a 0 to 10 rating scale.

Cognitive Status The Mini-Mental State Examination (MMSE) (Folstein, Folstein, & McHugh, 1975) was used as a screening tool to assess cognitive status. The MMSE consists of 11 items assessing orientation, recall, registration, attention, calculation, language, and praxis. Scores range from 0 to 30, with a score less than 24 indicating cognitive impairment. Those with a score less than 24 were excluded from the study.

Demographic and Medical Record Data

Background data included age, gender, education, marital status, religion, race, ethnocultural identification, previous pain, previous pain medication experience, depression treatment, occupation, living arrangements, and household income. Related medical data included type of surgery, American Society of Anesthesiologists (ASA) score, type and length of anesthesia, pain ratings and analgesics ordered and administered for the 24 hours before the interview, hematocrit, albumin, total protein, height, weight, length of stay, diagnostic related group, discharge medication, and activity restrictions.

Procedures

Institutional review board approval was obtained at each site. Data were collected in an initial face-to-face interview during hospitalization, and via telephone 3 to 5 days, 1 month, and 3 months after hospital discharge directly to a home setting.

Consents were obtained postoperatively, allowing for the inclusion of participants who had undergone emergency surgery. Potential participants were identified from surgical records. Nurses then were interviewed to determine whether the patients were medically unstable or whether they had experienced episodes of delirium in the preceding 24 hours.

Patients were approached about participation while resting comfortably. If patients consented, the BPI, GD-SSF, MFSC, and evaluation for self-perception of recovery after surgery were completed then or at another mutually agreeable time. Demographic and related chart data also were obtained at that time. Participants were given a copy of the consent form, tentative interview schedule, and contact information. A copy of the instruments was provided to decrease respondent burden. Reminders were sent before the 1- and 3-month interviews. Rehospitalized patients were not included in subsequent interviews. The following were administered during each telephone interview: BPI-SF, MFSC, GDS-SF, ESDS, and evaluation for self-perception of recovery after surgery. Research assistants received a standard orientation. The same data collector was used for the participants whenever possible.

RESULTS

The sample consisted of 192 male and female patients 60 years of age or older recovering from abdominal surgery, who were then followed 3 months after discharge directly to a home setting. Initially, 295 persons met the criteria. Of these, 192 consented, 84 refused, and 19 were missed. Those who refused to participate were significantly older than those who consented (mean, 75 vs. 71.2 years; $t = 4.28$). The most common reasons for refusal were related to the person's perception of well-being (too sick, too depressed, not up to it, too weak) ($n = 15$) followed by a desire not to be bothered ($n = 6$). Two persons withdrew consent during the initial interview; 13 subsequently had a change in discharge plans from home to another type of healthcare facility; 10 did not want to be bothered after discharge; 4 stated that they were "too sick"; 1 could not be reached; and 1 died. The remainder did not provide a reason. Eleven of the individuals were rehospitalized.

The age of participants ranged from 60 to 87 years ($SD = 6.8$). The sample was 46.9% male and 99.5% non-Hispanic White. The majority had at least a high school education. Specifically, 32.6% had one or more years of postsecondary education; 48.1% had completed high school; and 19.3% had not finished high school.

The most common type of surgery was abdominal aortic aneurysm repair (26.6%), followed by colon resection (22.4%), cholecystectomy (18.2%), appendectomy (5.7%), and abdominal hysterectomy (3.6%), with the remaining 20.3% categorized as "other." The average length of hospital stay was 9.6 days for the patients who initially enrolled in the study and 8.3 days for those who completed the 3-month interview. On the average, the initial interview was conducted on postoperative day 5 (SD = 2.2 days). The patients were categorized as retirees (79.5%), employed workers (16.8%), homemakers (2.6%), or unemployed individuals (1.1%). The majority of the participants were married (59.4%), followed by those who were widowed (24.1%), then by those who were single, divorced, or separated (16.3%). Those living alone comprised 29.5% of the sample.

The presence of a chronic painful condition was reported by more than half of the participants (59.2%), and this was most commonly arthritis. Home care services were received by 32.9% of the participants.

The means for the BPI and the MFSC decreased over time, and there was a concomitant decrease in the standard deviations, indicating that pain and fatigue decreased over time, and that there was less variance in the sample at 3 months after discharge (Table 1). Depression scores were increased at the 3- to 5-day interval, and subsequently decreased. The ESDS scores declined, indicating an improvement in functional status.

The participants' perception of how much they recovered increased over time from a mean of 57% recovered from surgery while in the hospital to a mean of 92.3% recovered from surgery at 3 months after discharge. The correlation between pain and depression was significant at each time point, ranging from .26 to .37, with the highest correlation for the initial measurement (Table 2). Pain and fatigue were significantly correlated at each time interval, ranging from .22 to .52. Fatigue and depression were highly correlated at each time interval, with the correlations ranging from .51 to .60. Functional status and self-perception of recovery were significantly correlated at 1 and 3 months.

The results of the multiple regression analysis with the variables entered at once indicate that pain, depression, and fatigue significantly accounted for 13.4% of the variation in functional status during the immediate postoperative period (3 to 5 days after discharge) (Table 3). The primary contribution to the variation in functional status during this period was depression. At 1 month after discharge, pain, depression, and fatigue accounted for 30.8% of the variation in functional status. Pain, depression, and fatigue were significant contributors to the variation in functional status at 1 month. At 3 months after discharge, pain, depression, and fatigue significantly accounted for 29.1% of the variation in functional status. Pain, depression, arid fatigue each made significant contributions

TABLE 1. Descriptive Data for Pain, Depression, Fatigue, Functional Status, and Self-Perception of Recovery

Scale	Initial Mean (SD)	3-5 Days Mean (SD)	1 Month Mean (SD)	3 Months Mean (SD)
Pain	39.93 (24.43)	20.86 (20.50)	11.79 (16.44)	8.76 (16.23)
Depression	2.97 (2.19)	3.27 (1.88)	2.17 (2.20)	1.79 (2.28)
Fatigue	47.58 (13.83)	41.45 (9.49)	39.18 (9.42)	38.42 (9.13)
Functional Status	—	30.82 (5.07)	20.17 (5.63)	13.84 (3.88)
Self Perception of Recovery	57.03 (23.30)	65.60 (19.69)	81.45 (18.63)	92.30 (12.57)

TABLE 2. Correlation Matrix for Study Variables at Each Time Interval

	1	2	3	4	5
Initial (Hospitalization)					
1. Pain	—	.37**	.52**	—	−.20**
2. Depression		—	.53**	—	−.09
3. Fatigue			—	—	−.20**
4. Functional Status				—	—
5. Self-Perception of Recovery					—
3-5 Days Post-Discharge					
1. Pain	—	.27**	.39**	.12	−.25**
2. Depression		—	.60**	.36**	−.28**
3. Fatigue			—	.26**	−.13
4. Functional Status				—	−.09
5. Self-Perception of Recovery					—
One Month Post-Discharge					
1. Pain	—	.33**	.22**	.33**	−.44**
2. Depression		—	.51**	.50**	−.50**
3. Fatigue			—	.42**	−.32**
4. Functional Status				—	−.50**
5. Self-Perception of Recovery					—
Three Months Post-Discharge					
1. Pain	—	.26**	.50**	.39**	−.24**
2. Depression		—	.54**	.43**	−.35**
3. Fatigue			—	.46**	−.34**
4. Functional Status				—	−.53**
5. Self-Perception of Recovery					—

**$p < .01$.

to the variation in functional status at 3 months after discharge.

The results of the multiple regression analysis with the variables entered at once indicate that pain, depression, and fatigue significantly accounted for 5.6% of the variation in self-perception of recovery at the initial measurement during hospitalization (Table 3). None of the variables (pain, depression, or fatigue) alone contributed significantly to self-perception of recovery initially. At 3 to 5 days after discharge, pain, depression, and fatigue significantly accounted for 12.3 % of the variation in self-perception of recovery (Table 3). Pain and depression made significant contributions to the variation in self-perception of recovery 3 to 5 days

after discharge. At 1 month after discharge, pain, depression, and fatigue significantly accounted for 33.2% of the variation in self-perception of recovery. Depression and pain made significant contributions to the variation in self-perception of recovery at 1 month. At 3 months after discharge, pain, depression, and fatigue significantly accounted for 16.1 % of the variation in self-perception of recovery (Table 3). Depression alone made a significant contribution to the variation in self-perception of recovery at 3 months after discharge. Diagnostics conducted for each of the multiple regression analyses indicated that multicollinearity was not a problem.

Pain medication was taken by 76.9% of the participants in the 24 hours before the hospital

TABLE 3. Regressions of Pain, Fatigue, and Depression on Functional Status and Self-Perception of Recovery

n		169	137	131	126
Dependent Variables	Independent Variables	Initial B	3–5 Days B	1 Month B	3 Months B
Functional Status					
	Pain		.001	.06*	.05*
	Depression		.85**	.84***	.44**
	Fatigue		.04	.13*	.09*
F			6.94***	18.82***	16.69***
R^2			.134	.308	.291
Self-Perception of Recovery					
	Pain	−.15	−.22*	−.35***	−.08
	Depression	.79	−3.23**	−3.01***	−1.31*
	Fatigue	−.25	.31	−.13	−.22
F		3.28*	6.24**	21.06***	7.83***
R^2		.056	.123	.332	.161

*$p < .05$ **$p < .01$ ***$p < .001$

interview, by 53.2% before the 3 to 5-day interview, by 28% 24 hours before the 1-month interview, and by 22% 24 hours before the 3-month interview. Fatigue in the hospital was not significantly correlated with hematocrit, albumin, or total protein.

DISCUSSION

The results of this study demonstrate that pain, depression, and fatigue are significantly related to functional status as well as self-perception of recovery in older postoperative abdominal surgery patients. The findings are consistent with the Conservation of Energy Model (Levine, 1991, p. 7), in which it is hypothesized that pain and depression have effects on energy and on structural, personal and social integrity; that fatigue is a manifestation of energy depletion; and that together they are related to a return to wholeness or functional status.

The results of this investigation are consistent those of others addressing functional status and illness from a more global perspective as well findings of studies focusing on patients undergoing specific surgical procedures in that pain, depression, and fatigue were related to functional status at all three data collection times: 3 to 5 days, 1 month, and 3 months after discharge. This indicates that interventions to address pain, depression, and fatigue are important regardless of the reason for hospitalization.

The lower contribution of pain, depression, and fatigue to the variation in functional status 3 to 5 days after discharge may reflect homogeneity of patients during the first few days after discharge. Surgical patients in general may experience a lower functional status regardless whether they have pain, fatigue, or depressive symptoms.

The proportion of variation explained by pain, depression, and fatigue 1 and 3 months after discharge highlights the importance of factors that have the potential for effective treatment during the postoperative period. Although pain contributed to the variation in functional status at 1 and 3 months, it should be noted that a number of participants reported that their pain at 3 months was not related to the incision or surgery, but rather to a chronic painful condition. Thus, patients with chronic painful conditions need to have their pain managed well to maximize their recovery from surgery. Individuals with chronic pain are more likely to have a subthreshold or major depression (Gallagher et al., 2000). The findings highlight the need to address not only the management of acute postoperative pain, but also chronic painful conditions to enhance the return of postoperative patients to their previous functional status.

Home care reimbursement has been limited in recent years. This is evident in that only one third of the study participants received home care services. Therefore, strategies to facilitate effective pain management after discharge, including the management of chronic pain, need to be addressed in the acute care setting.

The sample in this study consisted of patients discharged directly to their home, indicating either a higher level of functioning at discharge or a stronger support system than abdominal surgery patients as a whole enjoy. Despite this, depression made a significant contribution to functional status at each time point, indicating that the emotional component of postoperative recovery may be critical to the successful return of patients to their previous functional status.

Although fatigue contributed to the variation in both regression models, the t for fatigue was significant only in the functional status model 1 and 3 months after discharge. This may be related to the measurement of fatigue. Inclusion of ratings for the degree of fatigue and the degree of fatigue's interference with daily activities would provide more information and more direction for nursing interventions.

Pain and depression contribute to functional loss in older persons, which may be exacerbated when surgery is needed. Postoperative interventions have been standardized for patients undergoing certain types of surgeries with high volumes such as CABG or joint replacement. They are less likely to be standardized for low-volume surgeries. As such, there may not be the same impetus for attention to specific outcomes for these patients. It has been demonstrated that nursing interventions can make a difference in physical functioning and distress after CABG and ambulatory surgery (Ai, Dunkle, Peterson, Saunders, & Bolling, 1998; Moore & Dolansky, 2001; Swan, 1998).

The significant relation of pain, depression, and fatigue to self-perception of recovery in older adults indicates that healthcare providers need to consider their patients' perspective and their involvement in specific postoperative care regimens. Self-perception of recovery may be closely related to self-rated health, although research is needed to determine whether they are the same or conceptually distinct phenomena.

Pain contributed to the variance in self-perception of recovery. Therefore, institution of appropriate pain relief measures in the postoperative period, particularly in the first month after discharge, is important. Correcting misconceptions about pain medication and teaching patients about the importance of taking medication would facilitate the resumption of daily activities. Only 53.2% of the participants took pain medication in the 24 hours before the 3- to 5-day postdischarge interview. Efforts to improve pain management for patients who have chronic pain by incorporating an existing pain management regimen into the postoperative pain management protocol are suggested.

The group investigated in this study was not a random sample of abdominal surgery patients. Patients not discharged directly to a home setting were excluded. Some patients who declined participation or dropped out of the study indicated that they were "too sick" to participate. It is possible in the investigation of unpleasant symptoms that a greater number individuals experiencing extreme distress are not included. Thus, the participants in this study may have been relatively well as compared with abdominal surgery patients in general. Increasingly, patients are being transferred to rehabilitation facilities, skilled nursing facilities, and personal care homes before they return home. It is likely, but not known, that these particular subsets of patients have more extended postoperative recoveries.

A limitation of this study is that baseline data were not available because the participants did not complete the instruments preoperatively. Therefore, additional research including baseline data is recommended to describe the impact of surgery on recovery. The close relation of pain, depression, and fatigue to functional status indicates that a multifaceted approach including psychosocial interventions has the potential to enhance the recovery of older patients after major surgery.

Accepted for publication September 18, 2003.

Funded by the National Institute of Nursing Research, National Institutes of Health (1R15 NR04483-01) and an internal faculty research grant from the University of Scranton.

The author thanks Serdar Atav, PhD, Associate Professor, Decker School of Nursing, Binghamton University, and Therese Meehan, PhD, RNT, RGN, Lecturer, School of Nursing and Midwifery, University College Dublin, who provided consultation for this study.

Corresponding author: Margarete Lieb Zalon, PhD, RN, APRN, BC, Department of Nursing, University of Scranton, Scranton, PA 18510-4595

(e-mail: margarete.zalon@scranton.edu).

REFERENCES

Ai, A. L., Dunkle, R. E., Peterson, C., Saunders, D. G., & Bolling, S. F. (1998). Self-care and psychosocial adjustment of patients following cardiac surgery. *Social Work in Health Care, 27*, 75-95.

Baker, R. A., Andrew, M. J., Schrader, G., & Knight, L. (2001). Preoperative depression and mortality in coronary artery bypass surgery: Preliminary findings. *Australia New Zealand Journal of Surgery, 71*, 139-142.

Barsevick, A. M., Pasacreta, J., & Orsi, A. (1995). Psychological distress and functional dependency in colorectal cancer patients. *Cancer Practice, 3*, 105-110.

Benoliel, J. Q., McCorkle, R., & Young, K. (1980). Development of a social dependency scale. *Research in Nursing and Health, 3*, 3-10.

Christensen, T, & Kehlet, H. (1993). Postoperative fatigue. *World Journal of Surgery, 17*, 220-225.

Daut, R. L., Cleeland, C. S., & Flanery, R. C. (1983). Development of the Wisconsin Brief Pain Questionnaire to assess pain in cancer and other diseases. *Pain, 17*, 197-210.

DeCherney, A. H., Bachmann, G., Isaacson, K., & Gall, S. (2002). Postoperative fatigue negatively impacts the daily lives of those recovering from hysterectomy. *Obstetrics and Gynecology, 99*, 51-57.

Devine, E. C., Bevsek, S. A., Brubakken, K., Johnson, B. P., Ryan, P., Sliefert, M. K. et al. (1999). AHCPR clinical practice guideline on surgical pain management: Adoption and outcomes. *Research in Nursing and Health, 22*, 119-130.

Folstein, M. F., Folstein, S. E., & McHugh, P. R. (1975). "Mini-Mental State": A practical method for grading the cognitive state for the clinician. *Journal of Psychiatric Research, 12*, 189-198.

Gallagher, R. M., Verma, S., & Mossey, J. (2000). Chronic pain: Sources of late-life pain and risk factors for disability. *Geriatrics, 55*(9), 40-44, 47.

Galloway, S. C., Rebeyka, D., Saxe-Braithwaite, M., Bubela, N., & McKibbon, A. (1997). Discharge information needs and symptom distress after abdominal aortic surgery. *Canadian Journal of Cardiovascular Nursing, 8*(3), 9-15.

Inouye, S. K., Bogardus, S. T., Baker, D. I., Leo-Summers, L., & Cooney, L. M. (2000). The Hospital Elder Life Program: A model of care to prevent cognitive and functional decline in older hospitalized patients. *Journal of the American Geriatrics Society, 48*, 1697-1706.

Johnson, M. F., Kramer, A.M., Lin, M. K., Kowalsky, J. C., & Steiner, J. F. (2000). Outcomes of older persons receiving rehabilitation for medical and surgical conditions compared with hip fracture and stroke. *Journal of the American Geriatrics Society, 48*, 1389-1397.

Koenig, H. G. (1997). Differences in psychosocial and health correlates of major and minor depression in medically ill older adults. *Journal of the American Geriatrics Society, 45*, 1487-1495.

Lay, T. D., Puntillo, K. A., Miaskowski, C. A., & Wallhagen, M. I. (1996). Analgesics prescribed and administered to intensive care cardiac surgery patients: Does patient age make a difference? *Progress in Cardiovascular Nursing, 11*(4), 17-24.

Levine, M. E. (1991). The conservation principles: A model for health. In K. M. Schaefer & J. B. Pond (Eds.), *Levine's conservation model: A framework for practice* (pp. 1-11). Philadelphia: F. A. Davis.

Liao, S., & Ferrell, B. A. (2000). Fatigue in an older population. *Journal of the American Geriatrics Society, 48*, 426-430.

MacIntyre, P. E., & Jarvis, D. A. (1996). Age is the best predictor of postoperative morphine requirements. *Pain, 64*, 357-364.

McDonald, D. D. (1999). Postoperative pain after discharge. *Clinical Nursing Research, 8*, 355-367.

Moore, S. M. (1994). Development of discharge information for recovery after coronary artery bypass surgery. *Applied Nursing Research, 7*, 170-177.

Moore, S. M., & Dolansky, M. A. (2001). Randomized trial of a home recovery intervention following coronary artery bypass surgery. *Research in Nursing and Health, 24*, 93-104.

Mossey, J. M., Knott, K., & Craik, R. (1990). The effects of persistent depressive symptoms on hip fracture recovery. *Journal of Gerontology, 45*, N1163-M168.

Mulsant, B. H., & Ganguli, M. (1999). Epidemiology and diagnosis of depression in late life. *Journal of Clinical Psychiatry, 60*(Suppl 20), 9-15.

National Center for Health Statistics. (2002). *Health, United States, 2002 with chartbook on trends in the health of Americans*. Hyattsville, MD: Author.

Pouget, R., Yersin, B., Wietlisbach, V., Bumand, B., & Bula, C. J. (2000). Depressed mood in a cohort of elderly medical inpatients: Prevalence, clinical correlates, and recognition rate. *Aging (Milano), 12*, 301-307.

Pugh, L. C. (1993). Childbirth and the measurement of fatigue. *Journal of Nursing Measurement, 1*, 57-66.

Redeker, N. S. (1993). Symptoms reported by older and middle-aged adults after coronary bypass surgery. *Clinical Nursing Research, 2*, 148-159.

Rubin, G. J., & Hotopf, M. (2002). Systematic review and meta-analysis of interventions for postoperative fatigue. *British Journal of Surgery, 89*, 971-984.

Sheikh, J. I., & Yesavage, J. A. (1986). Geriatric Depression Scale (GDS): Recent evidence and development of a shorter version. *Clinical Gerontologist, 5*, 165-173.

Swan, B. A. (1998). Postoperative nursing care contributions to symptom distress and functional status after ambulatory surgery. *Medsurg Nursing, 7*, 148-151, 154-158.

Ware, J. E., Nelson, E. C., Sherbourne, C. D., & Stewart, A. L. (1992). Preliminary tests of a 6-item general health survey: A patient application. In A. L. Stewart & J. E. Ware (Eds.), *Measuring functioning and well-being: The medical outcomes study approach* (pp. 291-303). Durham, NC: Duke University.

Warfield, C. A., & Kahn, C. H. (1995). Acute pain management: Programs in U.S. hospitals and experiences and attitudes among U.S. adults. *Anesthesiology, 83*, 1090-1094.

Westerblad, H., & Allen, D. G. (2002). Recent advances in the understanding of skeletal muscle fatigue. *Current Opinion in Rheumatology, 14*, 648-652.

Yoshitake, H. (1971). Relations between the symptoms and the feeling of fatigue. *Ergonomics, 14*, 175-186.

Zalon, M. L. (1997). Pain in frail, elderly women after surgery. *Image: Journal of Nursing Scholarship, 29*, 21-26.

Zalon, M. L. (1999). Comparison of pain measures in surgical patients. *Journal of Nursing Measurement, 7*, 135-152.

Zimmerman, L., Barnason, S., Brey, B. A., Catlin, S. S., & Nieveen, J. (2002). Comparison of recovery patterns for patients undergoing coronary artery bypass grafting and minimally invasive direct coronary artery bypass in the early discharge period. *Progress in Cardiovascular Nursing, 17*, 132-141.